Play Long. Stay Strong.
A guide to help you keep doing the activities you love, for life.
More than what to do, it's how to do it so it works for you.
By Sean R. Robbins

AF824457

Published by Sean Robbins, Akron, Ohio through Amazon Kindle publishing service.

Editing, design and composition by LSI.

LIbrary of Congress Control Number:
2021919101

ISBN 978-0-578-98736-1

CONTENTS

FOREWORD

Why Play Long. Stay Strong.?

From the time I started my first fitness business, Sean Sports Training, I had thought often about writing a book. Fast forward several years after I founded Fitness & Sports Excellerated, LLC and I was still thinking about it. However, it was not until January 2021 that I took it seriously after a colleague helped convince me that I should do it. Sometimes it takes just one more word of encouragement to nudge a person forward.

I wrote this book to encourage you and nudge you to start and/or continue on your sports and fitness journey. In the book I share some personal, and hopefully, inspirational, stories about my sports and fitness experiences.

This book is not prescriptive---it is a guide. It can be read from start to finish or referenced from time to time. The information provided does not specify what you need to do, but rather how to do it, working at your level.

Your body needs your time and attention. We know that if we don't use it, we lose it. Yet, if we use it *too much* then we can lose it, too. As we age, we have to keep tabs on our bodies. It is different for everyone, but as we mature, we all need more care and maintenance. The sooner we get started, the better but it's never too late to start a healthy lifestyle.

I want to thank GOD for making this journey possible, all clients past and present for challenging me to learn and grow in my profession, and my family members and friends who have always been there to encourage me.

Play Long. Stay Strong.

IN THEIR OWN WORDS

In this section, I asked some of the people who know me well to write reflections of their experiences with me. I appreciate all of the thought that went into their reflections. In editing for length, I have maintained as much as possible of the original compositions.

When my son Sean asked me to write a reflection about him for his book in just a few hundred words, I knew it would be a task to keep it short. As the person who has known Sean the longest, I have so many good things to say about him. It has been my pleasure to raise him and watch him grow into the person and professional that he is today.

First and foremost, Sean was raised with a Christian foundation. He was active in church and at the age of 10 accepted Jesus as his Savior. He attended Sunday school, learned from the Bible and, among other scriptures, came to understand the meaning of Matthew 6:33 and Proverbs 3:5-6 as life guidance, guidance that he continues to follow today.

I knew that Sean was destined to play sports. As a baby he would sit in his crib and playpen and play. When we gave him a ball, he would throw that ball with such force that we had to take it away to keep him from hurting himself or breaking something. When he grew older, his passion for sports remained and he ended up playing basketball and running track in elementary school and throughout high school.

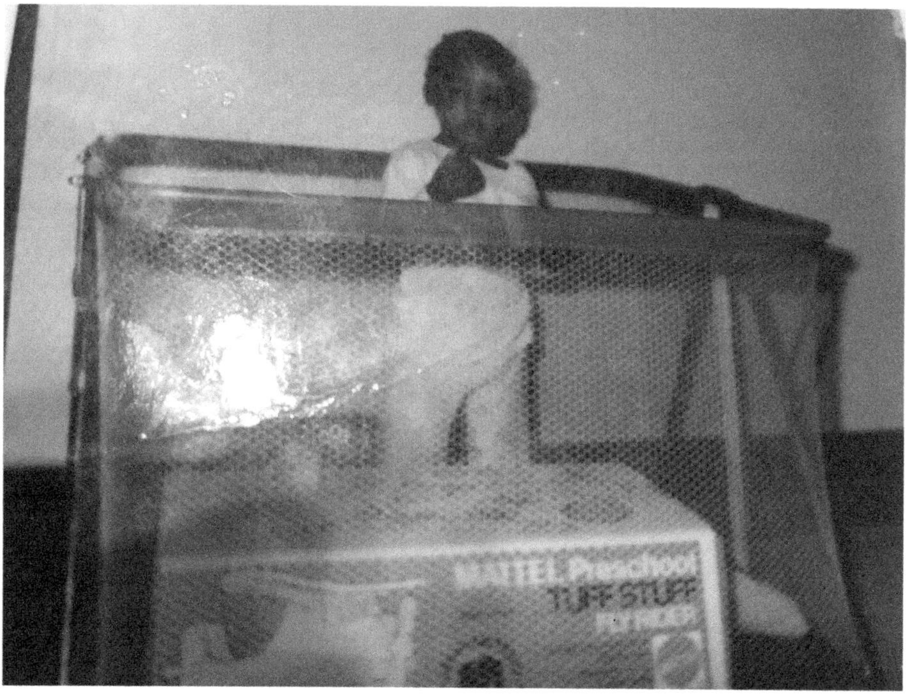

At the college level Sean's concentration was on track. After graduating from college, Sean became a professional in track and field and started traveling the world. That's when I got my passport! My late husband, daughter and I enjoyed going to see him at the various events, especially the 1996 and 2000 Olympic Trials.

Sean is a good listener and always has a positive word for anyone who needs it. Along with his love for sports and helping others, I was not surprised when Sean chose a career in coaching and training. Even outside work, Sean shares his fitness expertise and nutrition information with all of the family, including his wife, his stepfather, other relatives and me.

I must add that he keeps on amazing me as he continues to excel in other areas in the sports field. Sean's dad and sister Rhonda have passed away but I speak for the entire family when I say that we are all so proud of him and his accomplishments.

Dr. Betty Robbins March, Mother

◆ ◆ ◆

"Who is wise? He that learns from everyone." --Benjamin Franklin

When Sean invited me to write a piece about him, the above quote immediately came to mind. Sean is someone who learns from each person he meets. In my opinion, that's the superpower that helps him fly.

Sean and I met more than 20 years ago on a flight to Europe. At that time, he had just begun competing professionally in track and field and was on his way to a track meet in Russia. My husband and I were on the same flight, on our way to Amsterdam for a long and overdue vacation.

Poor Sean, with his long, long legs, was assigned to a tiny aisle seat in my row, and in a section of the plane with extremely limited leg room. Despite his physical discomfort, he did not complain. We began to chat about this and that, as many people do when they fly overseas. Mid-conversation, he pulled out a bag of assorted candy and began to snack. At the time, I worked as a registered dietitian and had just completed a sports nutrition specialization. I asked if he would be willing to hear some of the information I learned. He not only welcomed the details I shared during the flight, but we also continued to discuss and tweak his eating habits via email and telephone for months after. As a result of several nutritional changes that he made, his long-jumping performance also began to change for the better. Sean generously credited me with his improvement, but he was the one who did all the work!

That single flight launched a long and wonderful relationship that continues to this day. We share family milestones and celebrate each other's accomplishments. My husband and I even had the honor of attending Sean's wedding. I am thrilled that Sean decided to write this book. In it, he shares all he has learned, observed and personally tested---the secrets so many have used to improve their lives.

Who is wise? All of us who choose to learn from Coach Sean!

Dr. Janis Roszler, Author of Intimacy & Diabetes

◆ ◆ ◆

I may be wrong, but I believe that I might have been Sean's first "old bag" client. Despite (or perhaps due to) years of misuse, I was not merely out of shape, but relatively damaged. I had abused my body in various ways, starting with years of wearing three-inch high heels with pointed toes, 20 years of waiting on tables in cheap tennis shoes, years of sitting at a desk studying for a graduate degree, and lastly, owning and working on a 20-acre farm with 3 horses, 2 dogs and multiple barn cats. There is, of course, some overlap in these activities, and by the time I was 50, all physical activities had become very difficult.

My first foray into physical fitness was through a "Fitness for Women Over 50" program sponsored by a local hospital. I coerced two colleagues from work to join me in the gym of the defunct nursing college. I ultimately developed good back and upper body strength before the class ended and the trainer left. Next, I worked with a personal trainer at a local gym. My knees were pretty trashed so I barely held my ground on the exercise equipment. Around this time, I moved into a condo. When I didn't have the farm work (that doubled as exercise) anymore, my physical decline accelerated. But then came Sean.

I imagine Sean was baffled by my physical condition, but he dove right in with professionalism and an attitude of humility, and I knew right away that he was different. For starters, he called my physical therapist to get her input before designing new exercises and positions. He helped me to increase my arm strength despite weak, painful rotator cuffs. With Sean's training, I was able to do knee lifts, despite having no cartilage---a condition that kept my orthopedist hopeful about imminent surgery. Sean created floor exercises that strengthened my core, legs and back, without any pain or additional damage. It is now at the age of 76, and as the pandemic has kept me out of the gym for over a year, that I can really appreciate all that Sean did for me.

Over the years, I have learned more about Sean. I knew he attended Ashland University and had run track. In 2016, I mentioned to Sean that I had seen the movie *Race*, the story about Jesse Owens and his experience in the 1936 Berlin Olympics. Sean told me that he had broken one of Jesse Owens's records. I suggested that he take his nieces and nephew to see the movie and then brag about his record-breaking stat. However, Sean does not brag.

When Sean was inducted into the Ohio Association of Track and Cross-Country Coaches (OATCCC), he sent me a podium photo. That prompted me to do a Google search and I learned that he was a 1996 and 2004 Olympics alternate, that he was inducted into the NCAA Division II Athlete Hall of Fame, and that he trains NCAA and NFL officials. (He never bragged about any of this either.)

Although he would never brag about it, I know that Sean is also proud of his volunteer work with Victory Gallop. Recently I met one of his fellow volunteers and she commented about how nice Sean is to work with, his competence with the horses, and his compassion shown to the children in the program, two of whom are his niece and nephew. I have a few living heroes; Sean is on the list.

P. Marquette, FSE client

◆ ◆ ◆

I met Sean over 10 years ago, when I was looking for a personal trainer. In my opinion, his prowess as a trainer is unmatched. He knows right where to meet each individual and group he trains, and he provides challenging but varied workouts in every session.

Sean emphasizes the importance of variety in exercise. Switching things up like he does gives those fortunate enough to train with him the opportunity to learn, progress, and succeed. Great results are a natural outcome of the mindset and dedication that Sean encourages and instills in his clients. His strengths and success as a trainer are in no small part due to his kindness and calm, positive approach.

Whether he's working with professional athletes, high school students, young professionals, or retirees, his sensitivity to the needs of his clients is unsurpassed. His patient persistence and helpful suggestions to modify exercises makes continuing to train, even with an injury, not only possible, but rewarding. His endearing qualities are so appreciated by all with whom he works. I appreciate Sean for the training and his friendship!

Carrie Wagstaff, FSE client

◆ ◆ ◆

This is the story of how I met my friend and fitness mentor, Sean Robbins and how he enriched my life from a physical fitness perspective.

At the age of 55, I had surgery on my knee that required me to avoid bearing weight on it for six weeks. For most of that recovery time, I was at home, mostly sitting in a chair. Unfortunately, during that time I developed blood clots in my lungs and I was unable to work for six months. The clots stayed in my lungs for three months and, coupled with my weakened knee and legs, kept me from exercising and my physical condition deteriorated. I needed help getting back to a better level of fitness and didn't know what to do considering my weakened condition. Those were the circumstances under which Sean and I met.

Sean and I both belong to the same health club, but I had never met him. However, I knew he was a personal trainer as I had seen him numerous times working with other members. I had never worked with a personal trainer and, truthfully, I didn't believe in the concept. There was no way I would pay for someone to watch me do push-ups and sit-ups, all the while yelling "No pain, no gain!" Well, at that time that was my perception of what a trainer did.

I really needed help so I reached out to Sean and scheduled an evaluation. I showed up to the meeting with the idea he would demonstrate some exercises, and make sure I would do them correctly. However, our first meeting turned out to be different than I expected.

When we met, I really wanted Sean to know my physical limitations and what I had gone through during the past six months. He listened intently and I was sure that he understood me. Before he started to focus on my health conditions and exercise, his priority was to impart the idea and impress upon me that I am an athlete. He called *me* an athlete.

You see, Sean is over 6' tall, in excellent shape, cut to the core and has professional and street credibility. And to hear this former Olympian telling me I was an athlete, and that I should start to think like one---I thought he was nuts! He illuminated me by explaining that an athlete is anyone, regardless of age or ability, who takes an active role in maintaining their fitness and develops a mindset that fitness is a lifestyle choice.

Sean challenged my outlook on what it meant to be fit with the body I have and how it changes as I age, and to not compare myself to others. An athlete always prioritizes good health and puts exercise at the forefront of their daily activities. After hearing his motivational talk, I thought to myself, 'Yes, I am an athlete and now I'm going to start living like one!'

I love playing tennis and despite having flat feet and knee issues, I still play the sport. Before training with Sean, I would do an exercise only if I thought it would help me to play tennis better. Consequently, by focusing only on certain exercises, I neglected training the majority of my body. Sean helped me to understand that an overall fit and healthy body was the key to being a better player, and it would help me to keep improving and playing long-term. And of course, exercise benefits my fitness and health, not just my tennis game.

You may have noticed that I haven't written anything about the exercises I did with Sean. That's not because Sean's workout routines weren't excellent. They were, but the most important benefit of working with Sean has been the change in how I approach fitness as a component of overall health. I am grateful for my time spent with Sean; it has been life changing.

Norell P. Hodges, FSE client

◆ ◆ ◆

In January 2021 Sean gave a Zoom presentation on special fitness regimes for aging athletes as part of the Wisconsin Senior Olympics' (WSO) programs. The audience members were our participating athletes. Sean took some of the unique programs he's developed for sports officials and applied them to athletes looking to stay in shape and compete at the highest levels after the age of 50. We couldn't have been happier with Sean's presentation, as it was perfectly tailored to our audience.

Using the backdrop of Play Long, Stay Strong, Sean used his experience to touch on multiple novel ways WSO athletes can better train and prepare for their events. He answered questions thoroughly and with an eye towards helping athletes with their personal training and fitness needs. I was especially impressed with his approach in terms of using examples from his practice and extrapolating what works and what does not so others could learn from his experiences.

Sean knows his stuff, shares openly and is on the cutting edge of fitness. If you're looking for a topnotch speaker on fitness issues, he's your man.

Dave Simon, Wisconsin Senior Olympics (WSO) Board Member and Marketing Chair

Introduction

TRACK STAR

When I was recruited to run track at Ashland University (Go Eagles!) I enthusiastically signed up. I had very high expectations for myself as a college athlete and I am happy to say that I exceeded my own expectations. However, I believe I could have maybe done a little better starting out. Although I was blessed with the requisite physical skills and abilities, in my opinion I could have shown a bit more work ethic in training when I started but, fortunately, it did not take me long to adjust and become a focused athlete.

Looking back, I think most about the many ups and downs, triumphs, and defeats that I experienced on and off the field. Getting to the wins came at a cost: hours of focused, repetitive, and intense training and at times, some show-stopping injuries. The highlights and triumphs received the most attention from those around me---24-time All-American, Five-time National Champion---while the lows and defeats were mine alone to endure.

During my freshman year, I made it through half the season before I injured my left hamstring. It was a season-ending injury, so my coaches advised me to focus on strength and conditioning during the summer. I did what they suggested and returned in the fall semester ready to roll.

My sophomore track season lasted a bit longer but once again, a pulled hamstring literally swept me off my feet. One minute, I was darting off the block to the sound of the starting gun, running strong for 30 meters, 40, 50 with a national title on my mind then... *POP!* goes the hamstring. My coach, teammates and the fans in the stadium watched me stumble, hobble and then drag myself through the finish line. It was a huge disappointment.

So, once again, there was work to do in the off-season. That summer was spent following my coach's advice to balance the strength between my left and right hamstrings. I stayed on campus to get the extra training and to prepare for junior year.

My third college season was very successful, despite the recurring hamstring injury. This time, however, it was just a hindrance, and not a season-ender. I will call that progress. On to the final year.

Knowledge is the Key

When my senior year started, I had high hopes of finishing off my college career successfully which for me, meant a year without injuries. That same year, Ashland hired a new assistant track coach. Fortunately for me, the new addition to the coaching staff worked with me and helped me understand the reason for the recurring hamstring pull. According to him, it was from overstriding, and he taught me some techniques to overcome it.

For me, learning proper running technique was a game changer. That one piece of information stuck with me and, I believe, allowed me to compete for ten more years without ever experiencing another hamstring injury---even to this day.

During that time, everything was going great, from weight training and my improved running form to nutrition and timing. I continued to enjoy competing and my dedication to the sport never waned. So, you may be wondering, "Well, why did you retire from track and field when everything was going so great?" My answer: wear and tear.

Longevity

You can drive a long way in a brand-new car at a speed of 45 miles per hour, on a road with no bumps, no turns, and in perfect weather---provided you keep the gas tank full. However, at some point the tires will wear out, the engine parts will rust (need that oil change!), the wheels will need realignment and the transmission will fail. Every make and model are different so the sedan may run 10 years longer than the sports car, and the pickup truck might outlast them all.

Although our bodies are not mechanical, we are biological machines that require fuel, maintenance, and a well-informed, trained driver to keep us in the best condition for the long haul. This book is a guide for you, in whatever activity or sport you play and in the stage where you are right now, to keep doing what you love for your lifetime.

Play Long. Stay Strong.

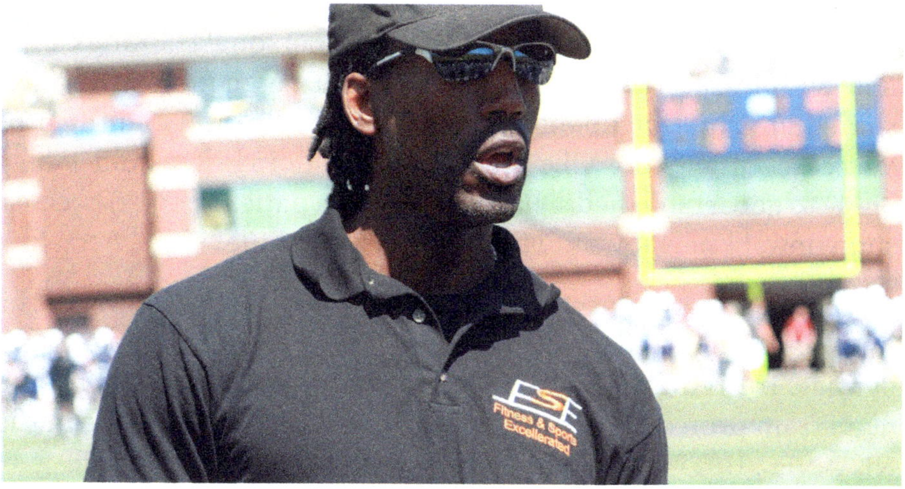

COACH SEAN

In mid-1998, I was nearing the prime of my professional track and field career, and I recognized that it was time that I started planning my next career move. I had a few years of college coaching under my belt at Baker University in Kansas, so coaching seemed like the best career choice. Plus, I was still competing so I needed flexibility in my schedule and I needed access to a really good training facility.

For a few months during the winter of 1997, I moved temporarily to Jacksonville, Florida to train. Getting away from the Ohio snow was an added bonus. During that time, I lived with a good friend from college who worked as a Personal Trainer. While I was in Jacksonville, the gym where my buddy worked doubled as my training facility. Sometimes I looked over to see what he was doing and I thought it was so cool that people paid him to get them in good shape.

I asked him a lot of questions about his personal training career and he told me that he thought I would be good at it, too. He shared information about professional certification and the pros and cons of the job. Like any job worth doing, it would take a while to get established. Thank GOD I am a patient person because somehow, I knew it would be the right job for me.

Within a few months, I had earned my certification from the National Federation of Personal Training (NFPT). With my credentials fresh off the press, I was excited to get started. My game plan: train professional athletes and help them rise to fame in the NBA, NFL, USTF, USTA and any other professional sports league. I envisioned myself smiling beside them with lights flashing as they accepted MVP trophies, Hall of Fame, and Athlete of the Year awards, or at the moment when they would be drafted into a professional league.

With those goals in mind, I contracted with Springside Racquet and Fitness (now Springside Athletic Club) to have access to space and equipment for my new clients. In the meantime, as I patiently waited for all of the sports agent phone calls to start pouring in, I was asked to facilitate a group fitness class at Springside. The regular instructor gave me some pointers to get me started but I was still a bit nervous, for a few reasons. First, it was a group class and I had never taught one; second, it was an Oasis class, a senior fitness class; and third, these clients were not the world-class athletes I had envisioned myself to be pushing to their max. Despite my apprehension, the class went well and the participants were happy. It was a good learning experience.

A short time later, I finally had my chance to train an athlete. There was a note in my mailbox from someone Pat (*all names changed for privacy*), who wanted personal training for competitive tennis. *Yes!* My thoughts were racing and my mind churning with all the plans I had for training this new client. I was ready to create the next superstar tennis player---someone like Venus or

Serena!

Did you notice that I had my plans set before I even met or spoke to the person? I had her name but nothing else. At that time, I could not search for Pat on social media sites to learn more about her. Facebook did not yet exist---*the founder was still in middle school*---and Google was just getting off the ground.

When we finally met, I discovered that Pat was a senior player, who wanted to continue playing at the same level (I believe it was USTA 3.5). I was not disappointed but the plans I had set for coaching her through plyometrics, sprints and running stairs would have to be adjusted. My new vision became to "make Pat the most fit and best tennis player at her level." Secretly, I wanted the other players to shake in their K-Swiss and Diadoras when they saw her name in their tournament brackets. I believe they did.

I worked with Pat for several years and as I trained her, I had to learn a lot about tennis along the way. Training a senior athlete did not fit my original vision; however, I realized much later that the experience was helping me to develop into the "super" trainer I wanted to be.

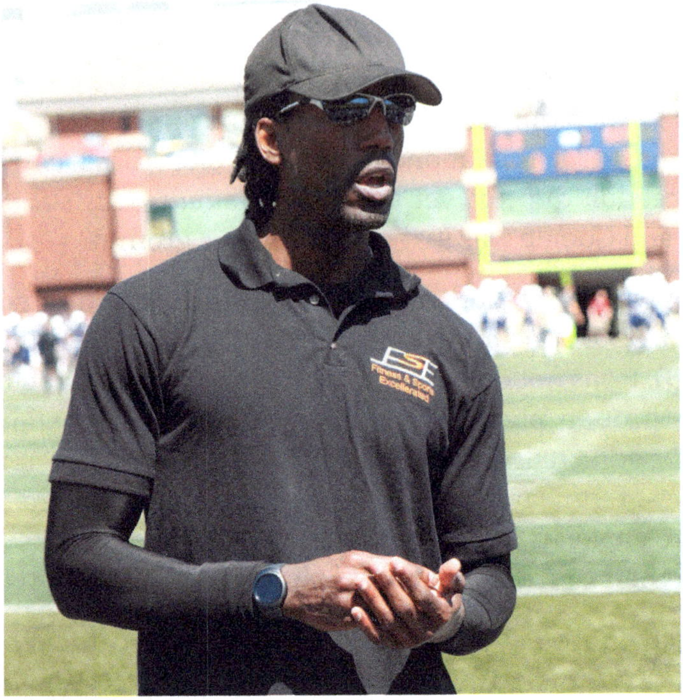

Coach Sean Robbins

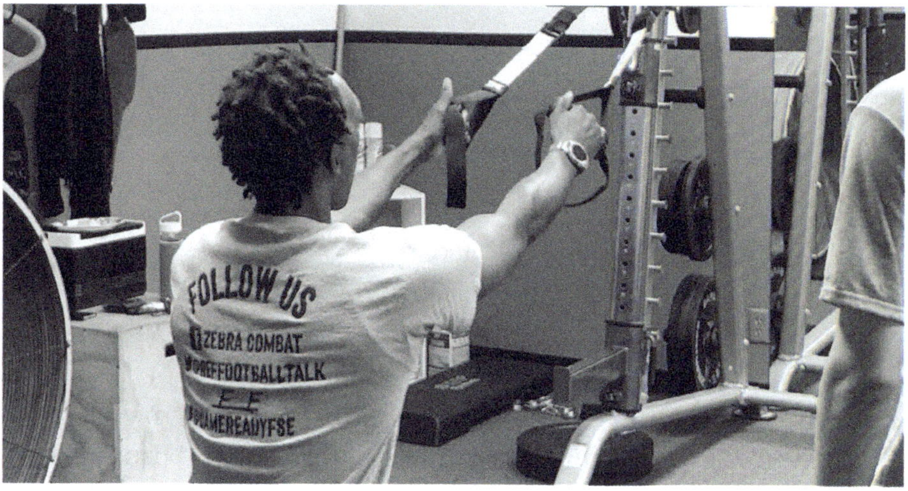

SPORTS AND FITNESS TRAINING

I am blessed to be able to say that I love what I do. I enjoy helping people to train their bodies in their current stage of life and help them to understand their sports and fitness future training opportunities. Publishing this book has given me the opportunity to reach more people and encourage them and provide guidance to help them to build the confidence and skills to continue on their sports and fitness journeys.

You have a vision to continue your sports and fitness activities and I want to help you reach your goals. Ready? Let's get started!

Play Long. Stay Strong.

YOUR SPORT IS BEING HEALTHY

What is sport? I define it as any competitive activity or game that requires skills, techniques, physical abilities and provides enjoyment to the participant. Whether you're training to be the best pickleball player or a champion NHL goalie, being competitive requires physical, mental, and emotional commitment to succeed.

Think of yourself as a professional athlete and think of your health, your life, as the sport. And like a professional athlete, you want to play your sport as long as possible. You want to minimize losses and maximize successes. You will do what it takes to win and winning requires that you stay in the game. The state of your health will be a major factor in what you can and cannot achieve in the long term.

Consider the importance of good health to our lives. The healthier we are, the better the quality of life. Regular exercise and the appropriate healthy dietary choices can help us to avoid negative outcomes such as chronic illnesses---illnesses that could impact us and our family members in many ways. Income loss, medical and caregiving costs, restricted mobility, and premature death, to name a few.

To me, being healthy means having the ability to do the things you enjoy. If you enjoy gardening, you will need to be able to lift the planters and bags of soil, till the ground, sow your seeds and later, harvest your vegetables and pick your flowers. You will need flexibility to bend on your knees and squat or sit low to the ground while planting, and then be able to get up. Although most people would not equate gardening to a sport, it indeed requires skill, physical abilities and it provides enjoyment to the participant.

Playing long and staying strong is a way of thinking. It does not matter whether you are a professional or amateur athlete, a newbie at training or an experienced fitness guru---the goal is to keep moving and doing what you love, whatever that might mean to you.

SEAN ROBBINS

DIY Training

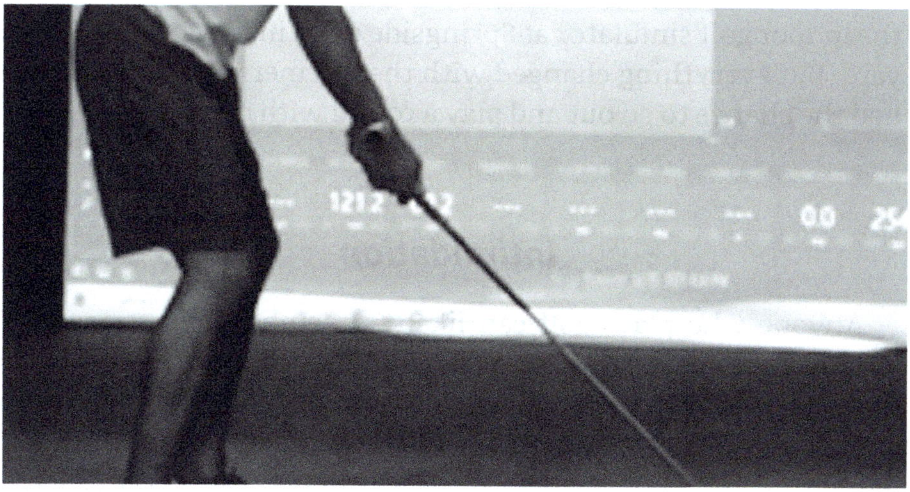

TRYING SOMETHING NEW

What's on your bucket list? Traveling to a city you've always dreamed about? Learning to speak a new language? Would you like to start hiking, skiing, running, or playing tennis? Or, have you recently made the decision to improve your fitness and overall lifestyle? Well, there's no better time than the present. Don't wait for January of the new year.

In 2020, the Covid-19 pandemic disrupted all of our lives in one way or another, and some were life changing. A disruptive change for me was not being able to play the sports that I enjoyed, such as basketball. I had to come up with something new to do and I chose golf.

When I first started learning golf, I was too busy to schedule tee times. I could only find time to hit balls at the local golf range, use the indoor golf simulator at Springside or swing away in my backyard. But everything changed with the warmer weather. Finally, I had the chance to go out and play a round with others. Yikes.

Intimidation

Anyone who plays golf can likely remember how stressful it was getting started. I never knew how difficult it would be to swing a club, maintain a stance and follow through properly. To not chop the club across the top of the golf ball and watch it roll five feet. Or, to keep the club straight and prevent it from slicing the ball to the right or left. To just tap it in the sweet spot of the club and watch the ball soar. Playing my first golf game, I was especially nervous when others were watching me. Needless to say, I can empathize with anyone who is beginning a new workout program or starting new athletic activities.

When some people feel intimidated, rather than shy away they choose to jump right into an activity and make sure they don't look out of place. That brings to mind a client, Jim, who was exercising with free weights for the first time. When I handed him a pair of 10-pound dumbbells to do bicep curls, I saw him glance over at a woman doing the same exercise with heavier weights and he said to me, "Those are wimpy weights." I held in my laughter and explained to him that we would use lighter weights to start to ensure that he developed the proper lifting form, and then add heavier weights moving forward.

Jim worked through the first 20 reps with the 10-pound weights. He ripped through 10, 11, 12, 13, 14...he started to slow down and his shoulders started hunching over. 15....16....17... By this time, his form was completely off and I asked him to stop the exercise. He looked at me, disappointed (and somewhat embarrassed) that he was unable to finish the first set. "Man, Coach Sean. I'm weak!"

Walk Before Running

"Don't think of it as being weak." I reminded Jim to have patience. Everyone starts with lower weights and if he continued to work out, then he would improve. It takes weeks and months--not days---of receiving and following instructions, performing the exercises correctly and safely, and a great deal of motivation and determination to find a sweet spot in exercise or sports. Working out with other people around you can be motivating, especially if you are a competitive person. Caution: work to your level and be careful not to rush through the process. You have to walk before you start running.

It's not always easy to start something new. The best way to ensure that you will stay in it for the long haul is to get started the right way. If you have any concerns, discuss your goals and plans with a health and fitness professional. Don't let intimidation get the best of you!

SEEK KNOWLEDGE AND GAIN UNDERSTANDING

At my middle school and high school, I played basketball and ran track. I even had a brief career on the wrestling team, but there are no trophies in that category.

My teammates and I were coached the standard way of the time: whatever the coach told us to do, we did it. Asking questions or complaining resulted in a two-lap run around the track, or suicides (racing to all the court lines) on the basketball court. When we were kids, challenging a coach's instructions was viewed as a disrespectful questioning of authority, just like in the military.

Those coaching rules do not apply now. Using military-style coaching was detrimental because it kept me and my peers from knowing the purpose of what we were being asked to do. We were pretty sure that the instructions we received were helpful, but we never knew the details of how it made us better.

It would have been useful to know that leaning forward during a sprint helps to conserve energy and reduces injury. I could have emphasized that technique to improve my speed. Or, if my coach had explained more about how power cleans made my legs stronger to boost my explosive jump off the board, then I would have been more motivated to do the exercise. Getting a good understanding requires good explanations and asking questions.

Leave No Question Unasked

As adults, it is in our best interest to ask questions and obtain as much information as possible regarding physical exercise. Questioning a physician or trainer before starting, during and after will ensure that you will have the information you need to prepare for and to perform an exercise correctly.

During training sessions, my clients usually don't ask why they are doing a particular exercise. They consider me an expert in my field and therefore, they trust that I know what I am doing. I appreciate their confidence in me but even if they do not ask, I will still provide clear explanations about what they are doing and how it helps them. For example, I explain how cardiovascular and strength exercises are necessary in fitness and sports.

Explanations are especially helpful when someone is spending a lot of time doing exercises but are not seeing the desired results. During the first session that I had with a new client, Connie, she told me that she had been trying to "get rid of this belly for years." She went on to say that she did over 500 sit-ups a day. She developed very strong abdominal muscles but the belly fat lingered.

To her, it seemed logical that concentrating on the abdominal muscle group would shed the fat in that area; however, I explained to her that in addition to targeting her abdominals, she would need to use an approach that included a mix of exercises for all parts of the body for endurance, strength, balance, and flexibility.

I emphasized that boosting her metabolism helped to burn fat, and that using the big muscle groups like the legs can burn more fat in the belly area. I explained that adequate rest and good nutrition were also necessary to get the maximum benefits of exercise and to recover properly. Having a more complete understanding provided her a new perspective on the overall training program.

WHAT WORKS FOR THEM MAY NOT WORK FOR YOU

Sara, a committed and somewhat experienced gym rat, was looking to recharge her workout. She wanted to try something new to lose weight faster. She read some websites, talked to a few people and even considered trying the grapefruit diet. Then she saw Mike.

Mike, a fellow gym rat, had slimmed down at least 20 pounds and the spare tire he carried around his middle had shrunk to a hula hoop. "You look good! What did you do?" Sara asked. He answered, "I'm a vegetarian now."

Mike went on to tell her about how he drank two gallons of water daily, ate a vegetarian diet, ran three miles, took spin classes and lifted weights throughout the week. Intrigued, Sara took mental notes and decided she would follow Mike's lead.

Sara made her grocery purchases and prepared her meals. She modified her exercise schedule to run, take spin classes and lift weights several times per week. After two weeks, she climbed on the scale and noticed that she was a few pounds lighter. Excited, she looked forward to the next week of training.

A few weeks later, Sara was still grinding on the routine but she was not losing the weight she anticipated. *She was not happy.* What's worse, Sara was not able to lift as much as she would have liked, and her recovery from her workout was slower than normal. She felt tired and was disappointed that things were not going as well as she had hoped. She was in a fitness slump.

It's not the diet or the workout---it's you

Sara believed that she could take the advice of her friend, do what he did, and get the same results. Her mistake was not taking into account her unique nutritional needs and physical capabilities. It is very likely that Sara needed to supplement her new vegetarian diet. She might have been missing vitamins and minerals that were present in her previous diet. Without a nutritional evaluation, she could not be sure.

Like Sara, it is easy for any of us to see the rapid weight loss, muscle gain or similar fitness gains of others and be seduced into believing that we can do what they do---especially if what we are doing is not really working for us. Before attempting to follow someone else's diet or workout, it would be wise to gain a full understanding of your physical condition through medical evaluations and perform research to find what works for you.

Finding Yourself

Keep in mind that we each have a unique body chemistry and a better awareness of it is beneficial to our health and wellbeing. Consider that some foods are viewed as healthy but not for everyone. One person could eat a peanut butter and jelly sandwich and it would be an excellent source of protein and carbs for weight training. Another person could simply touch peanut butter, suffer a severe allergic reaction, and fall gravely ill. A fitness routine can be equally hazardous if we neglect to get to know ourselves better.

Investigate and research. Determine what your nutritional and physical needs are. Find yourself first before trying to mimic what someone else does.

REALISTIC GOALS

As an athlete, you want to be the best. Being the best at any sport or activity takes a great deal of training and focus, and being #1 is not always in the cards. When I competed as a professional long jumper, I wanted to be the first to jump 30 feet. Hitting the 30-foot mark would indicate that I was the best in the world, since no one else had ever done it.

The unfortunate reality was that no matter how hard I trained, and regardless of how many motivational speeches I gave myself, I could never get past 27' 5". The fact that no other jumper had ever reached 30 feet gave me a little comfort but I often wondered, would it ever be possible for me? Well, perhaps with some performance enhancers in my system and an 80-mph wind blowing at my back but, ***no thanks***. I prefer to stay out of the path of gale force winds and taking illegal performance enhancing drugs was never an alternative for me. Yet for some, achieving an elusive goal is more than worth any risk taken to get there.

Competitiveness can sometimes drive people to make bad choices. Those who choose to use enhancers, steroids and hormones reap short-term benefits of bigger muscles and improved athletic performance, but they will pay a price in the long run. High blood pressure, circulation problems, hormonal changes and aggressive behaviors are just a few of the negative side effects of concern.

Others may literally beat themselves up trying to train for a marathon or cycling competition. Athletes may miss opportunities to compete because they are injured or too bruised to even show up. Putting intense levels of pressure on your body does not always result in a win.

Achievable Goals

Whether or not a goal is achievable for you depends on your internal motivation and physical abilities among other factors. Do what's necessary to train and prepare for whatever you are trying to achieve, physical or otherwise. And be patient because success does not happen overnight.

As important as it might be to you at the moment, keep your goal in perspective. Speaking from personal experience, regardless of whether you achieve the vision you imagined for yourself, it is not the only thing that you are destined to do in life.

If you make it, keep going. Keep striving to get better. If you don't make it, take time to reflect and change things up a bit. Maybe set different goals that fit your lifestyle, and abilities more closely. If you don't have the stamina, time, or resources to climb Everest or Kilimanjaro, take a hike up Cloud Peak or Mount Olympus instead. Just keep climbing.

WORKOUT VARIETY

It's easier to do the things that we are good at doing---or what we enjoy. In contrast, it is usually difficult, and less motivating, to do what we *don't* enjoy.

When I competed professionally, I always started my pre-season training in November. The weightlifting program was unique only to the pre-season, and that made it difficult since I would not have done the exercises for about a year. In each pre-season period, I also added new exercises to the routine to support my changing training needs.

I exercised for hours, lifting in the weight room, and doing sprints and plyometrics on the track.

Five-second squats, up, down! up, down!
slow lunges...bend, forward lunge,
weights...raise up, lower slowly
Frog jumps...lunge exchanges...sprint uphill!
(Feel the burn)

I grew to expect the daily sore arms and legs and overall muscle aches. However, after a few weeks of undergoing this self-imposed torture, it would easier and I would find that I was not so sore after every workout. I had gotten used to the workout, which meant that it was time to change it up a bit. By adding variety to my routine, I would adjust the intensity, prevent wear and tear from overuse, and stay motivated to do the exercises.

When you master a workout to the point where it becomes easy to you, you might resist changing it. You get comfortable and you want to stay there. Believe me, you're not the only one to feel this way! However, it is important to make adjustments to always maintain the appropriate level of resistance, and to keep your workout challenging.

Benefits of Workout Variety

Adding variety in your workout means doing different exercises that focus on different body parts. Jogging, cycling, skating, or playing basketball, tennis or golf are all good as cardio workouts. Mix it up by lifting weights to add focus to your hamstrings, abdominals, shoulders, and trapezius muscles on some days. Walk, stretch, do yoga, or practice Tai Chi to stretch and strengthen muscles on others. Run up and down the bleachers and sprint on the track for interval training. Do circuit training for a time-saving strength and endurance workout.

Adding variety to your exercises and the sports you practice early in life increases the probability that you will be able to continue those activities later in life. Doing one or a few exercises exclusively will increase the chances of wear and tear on your body. This is because if you are doing the same movements, using the same joints and muscles, it will wear those joints and muscles down consistently the more you play or practice. Doing multiple exercises instead provides balance of pressure throughout the body. Remember, the car driving at the same speed for miles on a straight road will, over time, still have wear and tear.

Variety in exercise has another benefit. The more activities you can do now, in years to come, you will likely be able to do most of those exercises, if not all of them. The reason is your body will have better overall conditioning.

A Little Math

Let's say you are doing 50 different physical activities or exercises right now. As you age---even with consistent training and nutrition---chances are you will not be able to perform them to the same level in the future. For example, maybe you will only be able to do half of the movements you can do now, which would be 25. That's still good! Or you might still be able to perform those same 50 activities, but with lower intensity or a decreased range of motion. Still all good!

But what if you are limiting what you do right now to only 25 different activities or exercises. Years from now you may still be able to do those activities at a lower level, but like most of us, you will do much less. If we use the 50% future estimation, then you might only be doing 12 or 13 of your current activities in the coming years. Is that going to be enough for you?

The point is this: building in variety allows you to do more now, and later.

Concerned about getting enough variety in your exercises? Work with a trainer to create your fitness program. Do as much as possible early on to prepare yourself and to sustain your capabilities for the future.

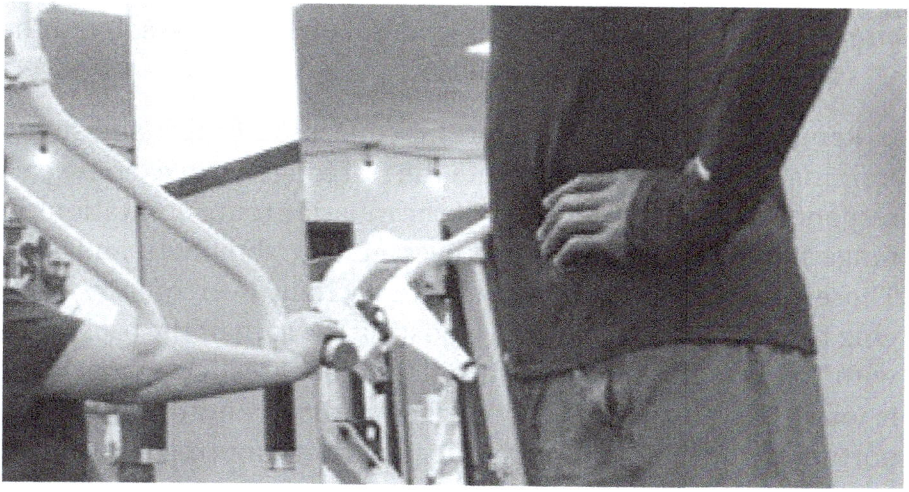

RANGE OF MOTION

I have worked with people of all ages and at different physical fitness levels. One client, Todd, a man in his late 50s with no sports background, hired me to get him started on a fitness program. The first exercise I demonstrated was the squat.

Todd got into position, bent his knees slightly and began slowly lowering toward the floor. Suddenly he stopped short of the full squat. He looked at me and said, "I cannot go any lower." Todd could not finish the exercise due to stiffness that prevented him from bending his knees fully.

This is a common range of motion issue among clients who experience joint aches and pains during exercise. Rather than continue to attempt the exercise and cause him more pain, I demonstrated a modified version of the squat, in which he turned his feet so his toes pointed outward, and he only squatted half the distance to the floor. Todd successfully completed the modified exercise without complaint. He was grateful (and impressed!) that he was able to perform a squat at all.

Range of motion is an important concept in fitness and sports training. The ability to complete the full range of an exercise corresponds to the full activation of the muscle group. Limitations in range and flexibility affect the knees, elbows, shoulders, and back. Those limitations can be managed or partially overcome by changing the angle of a weight lift, adjusting the arch of the back, or as with Todd, modifying a knee bend. In some cases, joint movement is restricted due to arthritis, or other medical conditions. It is important to consider your capability before attempting an exercise.

If you're looking for help in adapting your exercises, working with a trainer is a good next step. We'll talk about that in another chapter.

PUTTING TOGETHER YOUR PROGRAM

When I was an Assistant Track and Field coach at Ashland University, I put in many hours preparing individual training plans. I did not hold large group practices because I knew from my own experience as a collegiate athlete, that sprinters and jumpers had different needs. Giving them the individual attention helped them to hone their skills.

One jumper could only practice three days per week because he suffered chronic shin splints. His teammates and other coaches might have questioned this seemingly short workout, but sometimes you have to keep doing what you know is the correct thing to do for the individual.

Thus, we continued the program that fit his needs and I saw him progress as we moved forward. During the season that we implemented the customized program, he qualified to compete in the national championships, and achieved All-American status by placing in the top six at the meet. In this situation, the quality of the workout certainly proved more important than the quantity.

Do What Works for You

You have to find what works for you. You can find workouts and exercise information in books and in online material. You can even subscribe to video workout programs and sweat out whatever dance, aerobic, or resistance routine the facilitator demonstrates.

Do you know anyone who has purchased fitness training videos on CD, DVD or even VHS? How quickly were those materials set aside? In my experience, the novelty wore off pretty quickly and those impersonal videos were not ever watched again. The key word is impersonal.

Exercise facilitators who record a video or write a routine will never know when your ankle is hurt or be able to provide an adaptation of an exercise for you. They will not be able to recommend an alternative.

Now don't get me wrong; there are some materials that can give you a good start but putting together a program that suits you requires an awareness of your capabilities. Individual attention is important for anyone who has physical conditions or limitations. Do the necessary research and consult with health professionals to help you as you develop a training program.

If you are unsure about how to create your own, personalized workout program, check out the chapter on hiring a trainer. Having someone to walk alongside you in your journey will be worth the investment.

FITNESS JOURNEY: MAKE IT A HABIT

Have you ever heard that it takes 21 days to form a habit? From a fitness standpoint, I can only agree partially with that statement. It can indeed take 21 days to form good exercise habits---*if a person is provided adequate education and guidance*---and desired results can be obtained when that person takes time and makes an effort to put that knowledge to use.

Few people will continue playing a sport or exercising if they do not believe they are making any progress. The catch is that they will never achieve any results unless they keep practicing.

When I started playing golf, it was more challenging than I thought it would be. I was not hitting well, and I was frustrated. As an athlete, it is difficult for me to find that I am not good at any sport. Instead of giving up, I decided to put the time in to get better, even during the Ohio winter. I hit balls at an indoor driving range four days per week, and when I wanted to get a real golf experience, I practiced at an indoor golf simulator. As I continued to improve, I rewarded myself, first with golfing gloves, then a few clubs, a bag and finally a full set of clubs. Now I have two sets of clubs (yeah, I'm hooked). Introducing a bit of variety and some well-deserved rewards helped me to form my golf habit.

The same goes for anyone on a sports or fitness journey. It is an ongoing learning process. Setting small goals and celebrating your wins along the way will help to keep you motivated and moving forward. No matter what happens, don't quit!

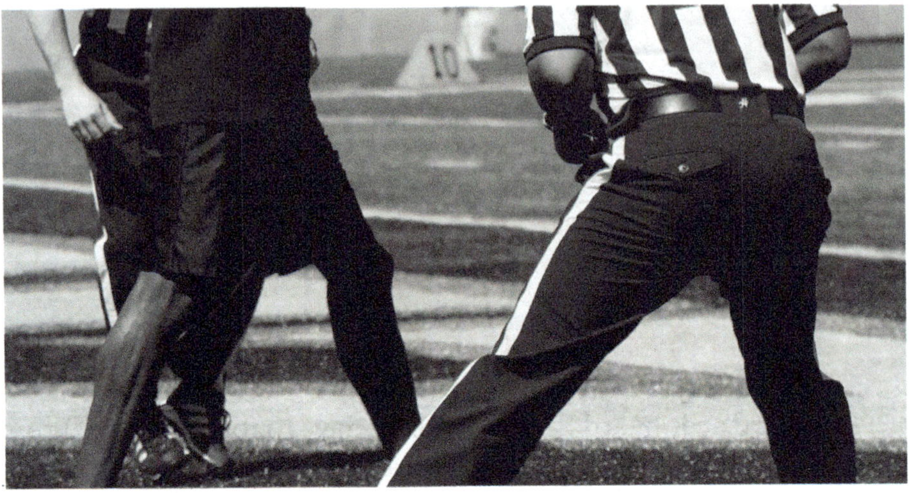

CLOTHING AND EQUIPMENT WILL MAKE OR BREAK YOU

The equipment we use as athletes can make us better, or limit what we do. When I say equipment, I do not just mean the aero climbing bikes, graphite composite tennis rackets, or specialized golf clubs--I also mean the simple equipment that can help in training and in competition.

Fully Equipped (or not)

When I was competing professionally, I traveled a lot. A LOT. In 1999, I was scheduled for a track meet in Brazil. Rio de Janeiro is one of the largest, most beautiful cities in the world and it was the host city for one of the most competitive meets on the international track and field circuit.

As a travel pro, I was always ready for the next trip. Like always, I packed my passport and visa (check!), spiked running shoes and uniform (check!), a change of clothing, including the essentials (check and check!). The first rule of the track and field travel circuit is always to carry onboard the bag with your spikes and uniform. I knew the route and all the restrictions. I also knew that all my flights after Akron-Canton would be on the big planes, not the puddle jumpers. So, I was also prepared with my carry-on bag.

My flight landed in Atlanta and I headed to the gate for the connecting flight. I was early enough to get a good spot in line. I walked toward the door and...

"Sir. Excuse me, sir?" I turned around and finally realized the gate agent was talking to me. "Sir, that bag is too big to carry on the plane." I looked out the window at the massive Boeing 747 and gave her a puzzled look. "Too big to carry on *that* plane?"

She explained that it was a very full flight and that carry-ons were restricted. "But..." I looked out the window again at the huge plane and looked at her again.

"You have to check that bag plane-side." I started to put up a fuss but decided it wasn't worth it---but it really was. I looked her in the eye and said to her very slowly, "Ma'am, it's very important that this bag makes it to Rio."

"You have no worries, sir. It will be there," she smiled confidently. I asked again, "Are you sure...?" as I reluctantly handed the bag over. Parting with it felt like I was giving up an arm or a leg because all of my competition gear was in that bag.

I was restless for the entire flight. Normally I sleep on the plane but that time, I was too anxious. When we landed, I practically ran to the baggage claim area--as if getting there first would make any difference in the time my bags would arrive. I waited patiently as the bags zipped by and the people around me celebrated seeing their bags appear from the magic door. You know the feeling I mean, the same as someone might celebrate the graduation of an oldest child or winning the lottery.

The sad news is that I never got to celebrate the bag's appearance and grab-it-from-the-belt moment. Continental had lost my bag.

My track meet was the next day, so needless to say, I was in a panic. I had none of my practice equipment. I was sitting at my hotel with nothing but my passport and visa, and the clothes on my back. I phoned my agent and thankfully, he was able to get me some spikes for the next day. I was grateful for them but since they were new, I would not have time to break them in. I scrambled to get a uniform, also never worn previously but better than the jeans that were doubling as warm-up pants.

As an athlete, I often had to push through whatever circumstances I faced that were beyond my control. In Rio, I refused to allow the clothing and equipment setback to stop me, but it did slow me down.

Unfortunately, in this case I did not perform well because of my equipment. The spikes had a higher heel formation (my spikes had custom inserts). The uniform was too big and uncomfortable, and especially for running. I knew I looked out of place and if not for the credential I wore around my neck, I might have been confused for a trespasser on the field.

The good news is my bag finally came. The bad news is, it arrived the morning *after* the track meet, four hours before my flight back home.

Shoes

In high school and college, I could wear any brand or type of shoe and think nothing of it. Basketball, running, high-tops, low-tops, sandals and flip flops...well, of course with the sandals and flip flops I had to move fast to keep others from stepping on my toes!

As we age, we lose the natural cushions (fat pads) on the bottoms of our feet. As that cushion diminishes, the ligaments and bones in our feet have to compensate and absorb more pressure. This helps to explain why, for some, it is harder to find shoes that feel comfortable to wear while exercising.

A few years ago, I facilitated a training discussion with a group of sports officials. The room got really quiet when I started talking about foot issues becoming knee issues, and knee issues becoming back and hip issues---what I referred to as the *injury domino effect*. The number one complaint from the officials was the foot pain that several of them were experiencing at the time. They had already suspected that the assigned shoes were the cause of their discomfort, and my presentation helped to confirm it. I took their comments and information back to their supervisors. It seems that they made a good decision to change the assigned shoes because the complaints have since subsided.

So which shoes should you buy for your training? If you are going to invest your money in some athletic shoes, be sure that you are considering more than the style and color. Just as when you buy a car, you will want to take that shoe for a test run. Strap your feet in and jog, jump up and down, and do some lunges. If they feel good enough to buy, you will still need to work out in them for a few days to get them broken in well. Some stores even allow you to return the shoes after a specific period of time before you make a final decision. Get the right shoes. Your feet will thank you for it.

Clothing

My experience in Rio taught me that having the right shoes and clothing can make or break your competition or training experience. You may prefer to wear snug or loose-fitting clothing, depending on the activity. Other than having clothes that are actually your size, before you buy consider the fabric material. Some good choices are dry blend, cotton or natural fiber blends that keep you dry even with heavy perspiration. Avoid synthetic fabrics that trap perspiration and result in stronger body odor. There are plenty of choices out there so do your research before you shop to find the best clothing for you.

Monitoring Devices

I am a techie at heart. Just ask my wife about my "techno trash" drawer that stores all my old PDA, cell phones, flash drives and other obsolete devices. When wearable health monitoring devices first came out, I happily made a purchase and joined the hordes of people eager to tell you about how many steps they had completed in a particular day.

I consider a heart rate monitoring device to be a good tech investment because it monitors the most important muscle in your body. You can use the data it provides to maximize your training efforts. It alerts you to changes. It can help you determine whether you are falling ill, not getting enough oxygen or are dehydrated.

As an example, if your regular heart rate is normally 120 bpm when exercising, but the next day it is 150 bpm (*and you haven't changed your routine*), then something may be off. It could be anything from over exertion, a cold or other acute condition. The monitor gives you one piece of data that might allow you to take action sooner than later.

Clothing, shoes, and monitoring equipment are just a few of the items you can consider as part of your training program. Choose your equipment wisely, and appropriately to help you play long and stay strong.

PRE-WORKOUT

When I was about 10 years old, my dad bought me a basketball hoop and installed it in the yard. I do not mean that he paid someone to install it in the yard; he actually excavated the hole, mixed the concrete, poured it, lifted the steel base and set it in. When it dried, he got out the ladder and connected the backboard and hoop. He was amazing.

After he installed it, he probably regretted it because my friends and I were very noisy when we played out there. All the neighbors could hear us bouncing the ball, hitting the house or the garage, laughing and shouting strategic plays all day long.

Early in the morning they would show up, knocking at the back door. Bang! Bang! Bang! "Let's play ball!" I would pull on my shoes and run out the door and onto the court, not stopping for food, water, stretching or any pre-workout activities---and not thinking twice about it. Today, if I tried playing basketball without some preparation, there would likely be some physical issues later.

Workout Prep

A pre-workout plan will not be the same for everyone but everyone should have one. I am in pretty good shape but the workout prep that I do now is appropriate for my age and activities. I do warm-up and stretching exercises to ensure that my muscles, ligaments, and joints are ready for what comes next. Most important of all, I have to eat something before I exercise.

A common question that clients ask is, "What should I eat (or drink) before a workout?" Like everything discussed in this book, it depends. It depends on your condition, training experience and timing of the meal before exercising or practicing a sport.

I advise my clients to consume the nutrition sufficient for their workout. What sport are you playing? Are you planning a short, easy workout, or a long, intense workout? A piece of toast may be enough for a short walk in the park, but maybe not enough for a two-hour tennis match. If you are not sure about what to eat, always seek advice from a nutritionist or trainer.

Another common, and related, question is, "How long should I wait after eating before getting started with exercise?" That also depends on the person, and the food being consumed. For people who are just starting exercising, chances are their metabolism is slow and it takes more time to digest the food. Working out too soon after eating can be uncomfortable and may lead to cramping. (*Do you remember your mom telling you not to swim too soon after eating?*) You may prefer eating lighter fruits and snacks, versus eating a heavy meal before exercise.

Keep the Fire Burning

At the other end of the spectrum is choosing not to eat at all before working out. Fasting during exercise is not advised. It can lead to, or exacerbate, health problems. Weakness and fainting are very common risks.

Think of your metabolism as the flame burning in a furnace. In starvation mode, your flame is anxiously awaiting some fuel. Adding exercise means the furnace is working harder, and without fuel, the flame is burning out. Feeding the flame ensures that it will keep burning and not extinguish when you need it, when you are training with weights, jumping rope, or running in the park.

Sometimes if I have not eaten for a while, or if I am pressed for time, I will eat an apple or granola bar during a warm-up on the treadmill or elliptical machine. It may be strange to see someone eating while working out but if your metabolism flame is calling for it, you have to respond. Grab your granola bar and sports drink or water and get ready for your workout!

POST-WORKOUT

What you do after a workout is equally important as the workout itself. If you work out multiple days per week, and you neglect a post-workout routine, then you are reducing your energy and recovery by 60-70%. You may or may not notice that you are operating at less than full capacity during each subsequent workout.

What can you do post-workout? Some recommendations:

- Do cool-down exercises. Lower the intensity, slow down as you finish the workout. Walk briskly or jog slowly for at least three minutes. Or. use the elliptical machine or stationary bike on lighter settings.

- Stretch your muscles. Stretch all the major muscle groups, focusing on the muscles that you trained. If you run during your workout, be sure to stretch your legs well. If you do bicep curls and chest presses, stretch your arms and chest muscles well. Hold each stretch for at least 10 seconds to get full benefit.

- Eat or drink a carbohydrate filled snack combined with a source of protein (a shake, chicken, turkey, etc.) within a half hour after working out. Take the post-workout snack with you so it will be ready when you are, and nothing will distract you from eating on time.

Do not just stop and walk away when your workout is complete. Incorporating the post-workout routine ensures you will maximize each training experience. **Enjoy the post-workout recovery shake recipe included with this book!**

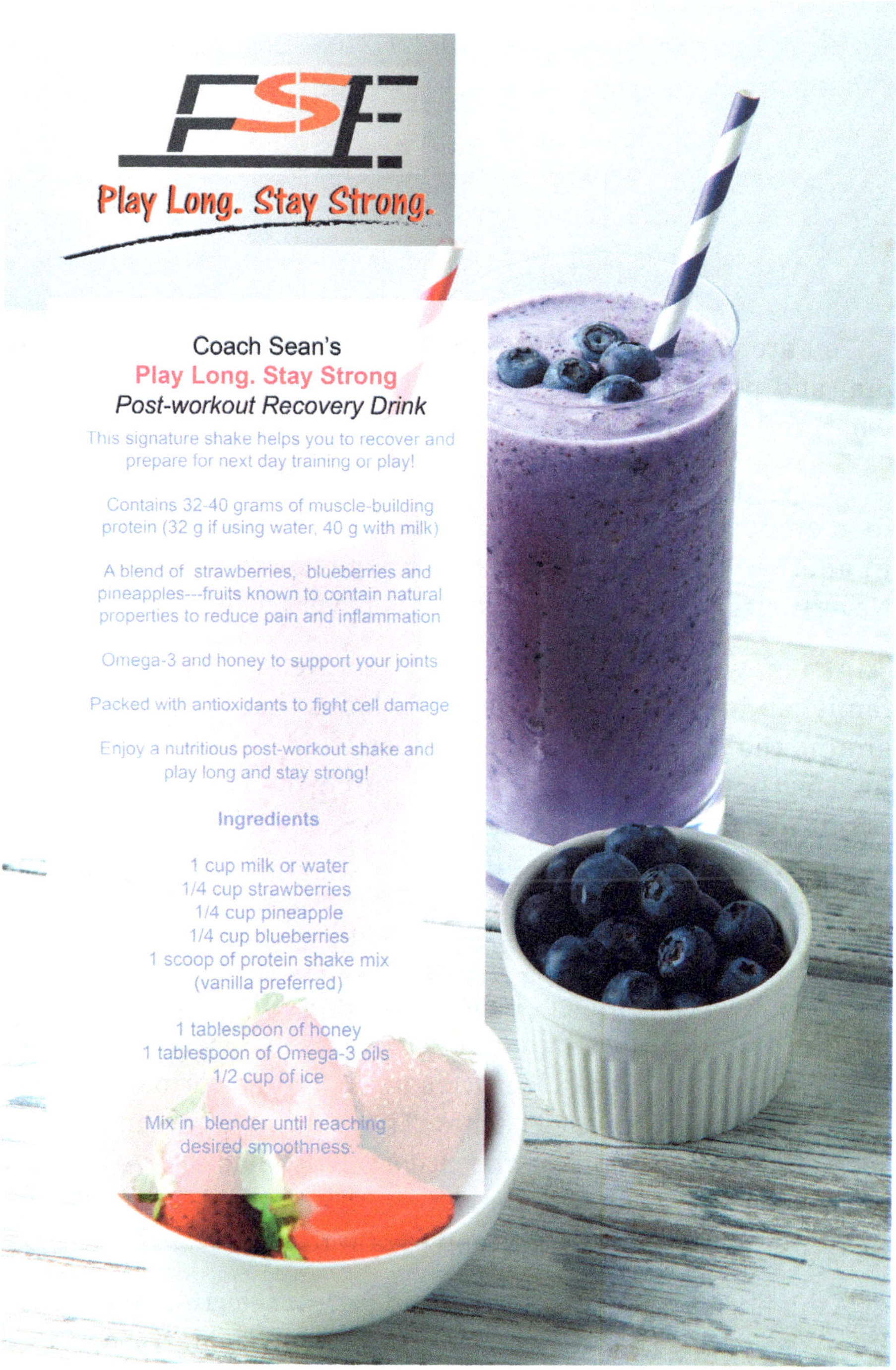
FSE
Play Long. Stay Strong.
Coach Sean's
Play Long. Stay Strong
Post-workout Recovery Drink
This signature shake helps you to recover and prepare for next day training or play!
Contains 32-40 grams of muscle-building protein (32 g if using water, 40 g with milk)
A blend of strawberries, blueberries and pineapples---fruits known to contain natural properties to reduce pain and inflammation
Omega-3 and honey to support your joints
Packed with antioxidants to fight cell damage
Enjoy a nutritious post-workout shake and play long and stay strong!
Ingredients
1 cup milk or water
1/4 cup strawberries
1/4 cup pineapple
1/4 cup blueberries
1 scoop of protein shake mix
(vanilla preferred)
1 tablespoon of honey
1 tablespoon of Omega-3 oils
1/2 cup of ice
Mix in blender until reaching desired smoothness.

GUT CHECK: NUTRITION

You are what you eat. Earlier, I mentioned the importance of pre- and post-workout eating and drinking. Now let's consider what, and what not, to eat.

In my "growing boy" stage, I ate everything in sight. My favorite food group included any cookies that made it into the cookie jar. In another chapter I have shared my penchant for Reese's cups. Nevertheless, at my parent's house, I ate very well.

As I grew older, my dad came to be a well-known cook in our family and neighborhood. He made foods that brought us to sit around the table on Sunday afternoons and holidays, and to nap for a few hours after. In addition to church, food is central to many of our African-American cultural events. All of the meals my dad cooked were delicious---including collard greens, chicken, beans, pig's feet, chitterlings, oxtails and other soul food delicacies---but some of these choices were not as healthy as others.

When I was younger, I did not think about food as being healthy or unhealthy. All that mattered was that I was fed and full. When I went to college, I learned some helpful information about good nutrition from my coaches. They educated me on the best foods for athletic training and fitness. I also had an eye-opening encounter with a nutritionist who further helped me to see why Reese's cups were not on the food pyramid.

Ashland University's cafeteria had a great selection of food and it ranked among the best in colleges around the country. As recent as 2018, the cafeteria was ranked among the top 25. I ate well at my new home and meanwhile, I grew stronger and faster on the track.

With a full academic course load, training and meet schedule, I did not go home as often as I wanted. When I finally had an open weekend, I headed home to see my parents and sister. Mom and Dad were happy to have me home and were eager to feed me. Dad pulled out his special pots and cooked up the finest soul cuisine of pig's feet, collard greens and cornbread, sparing no butter and salt. He muttered, "I bet you don't get this at your school cafeteria."

Although my diet no longer included those foods, I ate it to show my appreciation and man was it good! I am glad that I did not have track practice that day, or the next, because the heavy foods I ate would have slowed me down. I appreciated the cultural aspects of our food but I knew it was time to have a talk.

After eating, I sat down with my dad and explained that I would not be eating the heavy foods anymore because they were not good for my training. We had a discussion about what I ate and how I felt when I trained, and also about how some of the foods we were eating at home were not healthy for any of us---whether or not we were athletes. It was a difficult conversation because I was treading on the waters of tradition. My dad understood but I knew that he was somewhat disappointed.

Making a Change for the Better

I had made dietary changes for my personal and athletic well-being. My dad changed the way he cooked by swapping out some of the added fat and salt. He began to make vegetable and chicken soups, chili, noodles, and wings. He changed what he cooked but still kept cooking good foods and I appreciated his willingness to make the adjustments to create healthier versions. However, the one thing I asked him to never change was his barbecued ribs recipe! There was, and is, nothing like a Herb Robbins rib.

NUTRITION AND UNIQUE BODY CHEMISTRY

In my job, I get an earful when it comes to foods, new diets, and supplements. I have nothing against anyone trying to sell me on the super product that will give me an edge, but the usual response is, "No, I'm good but thanks."

As I mention in other chapters, we are all different so our training programs should uniquely suit us. The same goes for nutrition. To the extent possible, nutrition should be customized to an individual's needs and the activities that she or he is engaged in.

What works for some may not work for all. My go-to snack is peanut butter and jelly on crackers. I always have a grab bag in case I get hungry throughout the day. It meets my nutritional needs and provides the workout fuel that I require. However, some people do not eat peanut butter at all because it causes weight gain, which counters their fitness goals. Also, in recent years I have seen more people suffer from peanut allergies. Because of their body chemistry, for some people eating peanut butter can be life-threatening. We each must determine the foods that meet our needs.

The Three Questions

When my clients ask me what they should eat while they are in training, I ask three questions:

- Are you getting the results you want?
- Do you feel good?
- Can you maintain your new nutrition plan indefinitely?

Getting Results

The objective of a training program is to get results. More muscle or a leaner body. The shirt and pants fit a little looser. The check-ups or home tests show lower cholesterol, lower blood sugar and lower blood pressure. If the fitness plan or the nutrition plan is lacking, then you're probably not going to see the results you want.

Feeling Good

Do you feel good? You may be getting the results you want, but at the same time, you may be feeling tired, irritable, and *hangry*. Extreme diets may help you lose weight but the side-effects can be unpleasant.

Several years ago, I had a client who normally was full of energy. One day, we were working out and he had low energy, was breathing hard and was visibly fatigued. Yes, all of that is common during a workout but it was unusual for him.

I asked him about his sleep and eating habits. He hesitated at the food question, but finally confessed that he had started the Atkins Diet, which was very popular at the time. In case you're not familiar with that name, the Atkins Diet is a carbohydrate-restricted diet that attracted many with its promise of weight loss. Given his condition, that client would lose a point for question number 2: do you feel good?

Maintaining A Healthy Diet

Many of the clients I have worked with have been involved in sports that involve running and jumping. I have also trained with professional bodybuilders. When you see that title, bodybuilder, you might imagine a woman or man with bulging muscles, and bronzed, glistening bodies posing on stage with bright happy smiles on their faces. But are they really happy? Do they feel good? From conversations with them, the answer is usually no.

I have witnessed how bodybuilders prepare for competitions. For weeks before the competition they schedule extremely restrictive food plans (like dry chicken breast and an unloaded potato), and they do not drink much water. The diet makes them lean and mean, and improves their chances of winning. But then post-competition, they binge on the food and nutrition that they were deprived of. This is a diet specific to the profession and is not a diet that can be maintained by anyone. Zero points for question three.

The goal is to have balance and not deprive yourself. Do your research and try variety in your food plan and find what works for you.

A Note About Eliminating Trigger Foods

Completely giving up sweet snacks, fries and burgers is great for your waistline and many health conditions, but is it realistic? For most people, gradually reducing consumption is a better method compared to giving everything up cold-turkey. Otherwise, you might find yourself going back to the trigger foods in moments of weakness. Trust me, I know.

In college, I ate ice cream so often that the servers could have my order prepared before I reached the counter. Instead of eating ice cream every day, I began eating it every other day, then not buying it every week until I have reached the point now where I eat it infrequently. I enjoy ice cream when I have it but I don't crave it as I did in the past. You can make the changes to your diet; just do it at your own pace.

Hydration

Good hydration matters. Water is an essential element of nutrition that must not be overlooked, especially when in training. If you have ever experienced the pain of a nighttime charley horse, then you know what I mean. It is not common that professional athletes neglect their water intake, but it happens.

At the 1996 Olympic Trials in Atlanta, I remember that it was over 100 degrees on the track and everyone was perspiring, losing water to the air. Most of us were taking periodic sips of water and sports drinks. I waited on deck for the jumper ahead of me to take his turn on the runway. I could hear his family in the crowd shouting words of encouragement. "Go for it!" "You can do this; you've worked so hard!" I am pretty sure I heard someone yell, "You've got bills to pay!"

The jumper started running towards the pit, but after a few steps, one of his legs cramped and he fell hard to the ground. He did not drink enough water. The good news is, he did not make the same mistake twice. When I saw him again, it was at the 2000 Olympic trials. That day, he was carrying around a gallon jug of water like it was part of his body.

For most people without health conditions, being able to answer yes to all three nutrition questions indicates that you have a good plan. If you are unsure, speak to your physician, get expert advice from a trainer or nutritionist, and research to find information about the nutritional needs of your sport or activity. Stay healthy and hydrated to stay in the game.

SEAN ROBBINS

Finding your Balance: Nutrition

GYM RATS AND HEALTH FOOD NUTS

Some people will spend all day in the gym or sweating for hours on a field, and when they are finished, they will then eat the unhealthiest foods imaginable. Then, there are others who meticulously choose their foods at the health food stores, boil, steam, and bake (never fry!) but choose to never set foot in a gym or exercise. As you probably already know, being a gym rat doesn't make you the healthiest person if you neglect nutrition, and conversely, good nutrition alone is not enough either. Having balance---getting adequate sleep, a healthy diet, and regular exercise---is key for a healthy lifestyle.

Whether it is our sleep schedule, eating habits or exercise, we are only as strong as our weakest link. One of my strategies is to identify my clients' weakest links and then work with them to make the necessary adjustments.

Some clients have complained about feeling tired or gaining weight unexpectedly. I ask questions and some confess that they are staying up late to binge watch a favorite show, or that they went back for seconds of the chocolate ice cream or another tasty dessert. Believe me, I understand...I like ice cream too!

Eating Right

When I was in high school, my diet consisted of almost 100% junk food during the day. I ate donut sticks, French fries, Reese's cups and drank all kinds of sugary drinks. I had so many Reese's wrappers that I started collecting them and stuffing them between the pages of my history book, and eventually they broke the binding. Thankfully, my parents never found out about my lunches and it was fortunate for me, they were feeding me healthy breakfasts and balanced dinners to offset my daytime junk food addictions.

As a teenager, I could get away with eating like that and still perform well in basketball and track. However, I do regret my food choices and I wonder how much better I would have been then, and now, if I had opted for a more nutritional diet.

Today, there is no way I could eat so much junk food and maintain my fitness level. My body has changed over time and I take better care of myself. I sleep more, avoid alcohol, exercise five days per week, drink water instead of pop (that's soda for you southerners) and I eat healthier meals. I have adjusted more and more as I have aged. But in case you're wondering, yes, I still eat the Reese's cups---but just not as often.

Making the right choices about what you eat is half of the story. Much of this book is dedicated to ideas about how to maximize your training experience. The takeaway from this section is not to focus on either diet or exercise, but to find a balance to achieve the results you want.

SEEING RESULTS

Seeing the results you want. It's why we do what we do: lifting weights at the fitness center, cycling on the trails, avoiding the enticing milkshake, walking the track, eating more broccoli and carrots than chocolate covered raisins, or doing aerobic exercises in our homes. We make the right choices.

Results Vary Depending on Lifestyle and the Individual. Results can mean different things to different people. Being able to exercise with little or no pain, and still be able to complete everyday tasks. Walking and climbing stairs without assistance. Hearing a physician confirm improved numbers after a panel of tests. Running a mile.

For many people, the fitness goal is to have a lean, muscular body with six-pack abs. Although that body style is achievable (if you put the work in!), your actual results will vary according to your physical capabilities, nutritional needs and lifestyle. Results also depend on your activity and sport.

The abilities to squat, lift objects and bend over are important to gardeners. For golfers, maintaining flexibility and shoulder and back strength are essential. Consider your capabilities as you set your goals. Make sure your fitness training is appropriate for you, so you will be able to start, and continue, doing the activities and sports that you enjoy.

Don't Judge a House by its Façade

What a fabulous house! We have all driven past a house that was so stunning that we had to slow down to take it all in. But the outer appearance may belie what is behind the beautiful building and the landscaping in the front yard. There may be plumbing issues. The house might have cracks in the foundation. The roof may leak. The same can be said for people we see who are thin or have other characteristics typically associated with being the picture of health.

People come in many shapes and sizes and being physically fit takes on a different appearance depending on genetics, race, and gender. In other words, there is no standard body type. Obsessing over an external appearance that may not fit with a person's body type can lead to choices that are detrimental to one's health.

Getting to Your Results

Because looks can be deceiving, having good health is the gold standard and that is the target that we all should aim for. Before setting goals and taking the steps to improve your health, be aware of your physical condition and capabilities. Also, consider your family and social environments that can help or hinder you.

Physical condition

Get the exams and tests that will inform you about your current condition. Blood pressure, cholesterol, vitamins and minerals, endurance tests and analyses will identify your weaknesses and areas for improvement. Know your plumbing!

Physical Abilities

Assess what you can and cannot do. Learn this with the help of a physician and/or trainer. Whether it is a competitive sport, low-impact walking, or home gardening, get to know your current ability and move forward.

At-home Habits

Make good health and fitness a family value. The more that your family supports or shares your healthy lifestyle goals, the more successful you will be. Get everyone at home involved with the shopping, cooking and daily fitness and exercise plans. And, parents, do not allow your children to make bad food choices now. Get them started on a healthy path.

Social Networks

As with family ties, the people you spend time with on a regular basis will influence how closely you stick to your plan. If your favorite places to hang out with friends are restaurants, choose restaurants that offer healthy meal choices. Or skip the restaurant entirely and head for the park. Hang out with people who share your health and wellness goals.

Take ownership of your health and wellness results. Make sure your expectations for fitness results are not based on what you see others achieve but are appropriate to your physical fitness and lifestyle. You are uniquely designed and equipped to reach your highest potential.

Hire A Trainer

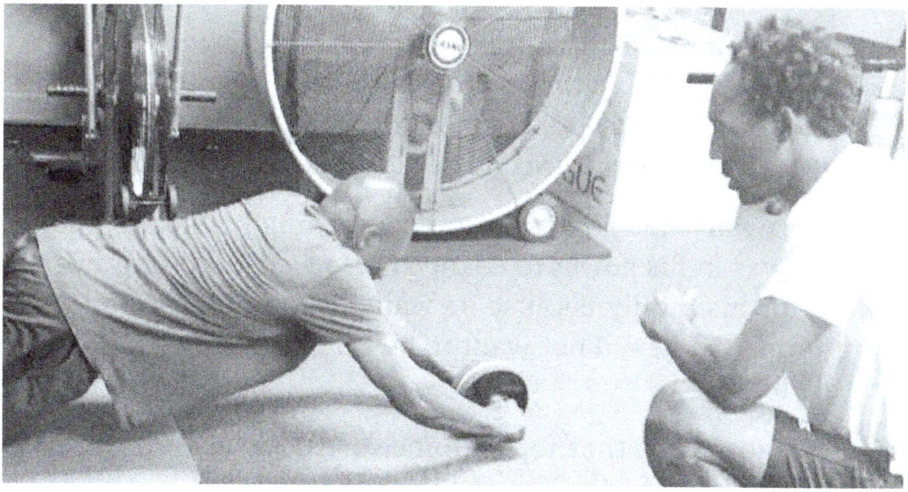

DON'T BE AFRAID TO ASK FOR HELP

I have observed that some people will keep putting off exercise for a long time. Their reasons for delaying are valid. The most common is a lack of time because of family and work responsibilities. What gets their attention is a decline in their physical condition, coupled sometimes by explicit warnings from a physician.

Everyone reacts to doctor's warnings differently. Some take immediate action. Others feel helplessness, which can turn into despair if they further delay taking action. That can happen if they believe that any improvement or recovery will require a huge undertaking. The time and effort required will come at a great cost---but inaction at an even greater cost.

Take the Step to Get Help

A club member, Tim, called me to express interest in training. He told me about his situation and what he was hoping to do. He described himself as very overweight, busy, somewhat stressed and he realized that it was time he did something about it.

Tim saw an undesirable future concerning his health and he knew it was in his power to change it. He wanted to improve his health for his family because he wanted to be around for them long-term, and he did not want to be a burden on them if he fell gravely ill.

I thought about that for a moment. That was a very selfless way of thinking. I told Tim that I appreciated his honesty and looked forward to training him.

We set up an appointment for the first Monday in April, at 5:00 p.m. I stood in the lobby waiting, looking around for a new face, and greeted the regular members at the busiest time of day. All of the adults and some school kids milled around talking and laughing at the pre-workout, non-alcoholic happy hour.

Tim waved as he came in, appearing enthusiastic and ready to get started. I saw his expression change slightly as he glanced at the crowd. Uh-oh---I thought to myself---this group of people might be a little intimidating...

A Little Nudge

Whether it was the frustration with the weight he was trying to lose, or nervousness about the number of people in the crowd, I recognized that look of concern. I walked over to Tim, shook his hand, and did my best to put him at ease. "Ready to get started?" And off we went.

We walked to an area in a corner of the first floor to do the physical assessment. We were working in a spot where there would be very little foot traffic, and it was out of the view of most members. That seemed to put Tim at ease.

After the initial assessment, we spent time on exercises that would build Tim's confidence on the first day. I set some achievable goals, which he quickly met, and we discussed goals that he would need to work at and meet over time.

To encourage him, I let him know that he was not alone in this fitness journey and everybody in the lobby that evening had also had a first day at the gym. What seemed to really encourage him were comments I made about some of my other clients working out nearby.

"See that lady over on the treadmill? She has lost over 50 pounds since she started coming here."

"The guy over on the leg press? He lost 30 pounds and started playing tennis."

"Stick with me and someday I will point you out to another client on her or his first day."

An important part of a trainer's job is to make sure clients feel comfortable in the gym, or wherever the training takes place. For some clients, it is a huge step to ask for help and show up; gym intimidation is an easy way to lose them. In Tim's case, I was familiar with the expression he wore on his face and the first-day-of-training butterflies. His level of comfort and encouragement that first day was an important factor for him coming back to the gym to train with me, and then later on his own.

GET HELP EARLY

Don't wait until you're desperate to make a change. We like to say that it's never too late to get started, but it is better to address a problem proactively, or nip it in the bud once you become aware of it. If you don't feel like you can do it on your own, and know you could use some help, start by getting advice from your medical team. Contact a local fitness facility and interview some trainers. Talk to friends and relatives who exercise regularly. Go online and watch videos. Regardless of how you do it, just get started and do not be afraid to ask someone for help.

What a Trainer Can Do for You

What can you expect from a trainer? Well, that depends on your goals and what you are training to be able to do. In general, your trainer is the person who provides guidance and direction---a coach and a mentor. Having good communication and setting clear expectations will be essential to forging a successful relationship, whether short or long-term. The process that I follow with clients is constructed with the objectives of keeping clients informed and measuring progress toward their goals.

Here's an overview of what that might look like:

- Introduction. A phone call or in-person meeting with a potential client. It is a brief discussion about training, goals, expectations, restrictions, and current physical status.

- Scheduling. Compare schedules and set up the initial appointment and location.

- First Day of Training. From the warm-up and to the final stretching, the first session is a benchmarking or baselining session. We recap goals as I walk the client through a training routine. I ask questions and monitor for pain or discomfort. We discuss future training sessions.
- Training Session 2+. During ongoing training, clients share their motivations, strengths and weaknesses and I support and encourage them. I gage their capabilities and watch for indications of irritation or injury. I give them achievable challenges for a particular day and set stretch goals over the next several sessions. As the client gets more comfortable training with me, she or he will share more information about their health and habits, information that I use to present relevant fitness education, and in developing the overall training plan.
- Workout Plan. Some clients prefer to have one-on-one individual attention or work with a trainer in pairs of clients who have the same fitness goals. Others may want to work out on their own. In all situations, I create workout plans specific to the client requirements. This type of plan incorporates information about physical condition, general health and wellness, nutrition, scheduling, and physical information gathered during my time with them.

Two Minds are Often Better Than One

Your trainer is your coach who is there to propel you to your goals, whatever they might be. Consider working with someone to help you on your fitness journey, at the start or for its entirety.

Injury: More Pain. No Gain.

"No matter how bad it hurts, I have to keep going to win."

PLAYING THROUGH THE PAIN

If you have been watching gymnastics long enough, you may recall Dianne Durham's struggle with an ankle injury. According to ESPN, she was Bela Karolyi's first elite athlete in the United States. Dianne's injury sat her down during the 1984 U.S. trials, and she missed her chance for the Summer Olympics. She walked away from the trials on crutches.

You may also remember seeing gymnast Kerri Strug, who was also suffering an ankle injury during high-stakes competition. She completed a vault that secured the U.S. team a gold medal win in the 1996 Olympics. She was injured and carried away from the floor immediately after competing.

Both athletes had the same coach, and both had ankle injuries. They both also retired shortly after their injuries. The only difference is that one left in a blaze of televised glory, and the other left quietly without a victory. That is the reason you may know one and not the other.

At some point all of us experience pain---emotional or physical. Culturally, we are taught to push through the pain. *No pain, no gain*---the phrase used to encourage mental and physical toughness---is repeated from locker rooms, training fields and courts around the country to motivate people to keep going, to get the glory. I understand this concept well because of my own experience of being injured before the 2000 Olympic Trials.

Ignoring pain in the quest for gain is not always good. Have you ever sprained your ankle running and tried to keep going? I recommend instead that if you experience pain, change what you're doing, how much you do, or how you do it---but don't ignore it or try to play through because it may get worse over time.

Training is often cut short when people experience pain or have an injury. Now, I am not referring to muscle soreness or stiffness after a heavy workout, but rather persistent pain. As a sports and fitness trainer, my objective is to ensure that my clients reach their goals safely, effectively and with minimal pain or discomfort. I am fairly certain that I have annoyed my clients by frequently asking, "Do you feel any pain?" Different people have different pain thresholds so I make it a point to explain that if there is pain that it does not necessarily mean that we will have to stop the exercise.

Pain Is Not a Sign of Weakness or Failure

Regardless of what you learned growing up, what you have heard athletes say or watched them do, bearing pain during sports or fitness training does not determine how tough you are. Nor does it indicate weakness or failure. Pain is the body's early warning system. Don't ignore it. Take the necessary steps to address it so you can stay in the game.

Overcoming Physical Setbacks

I had missed my chance to be a member of the 1996 U.S. Olympic team by a few centimeters at trials and I was confirmed as an alternate. So, I had something to prove at the 2000 trials in Sacramento. Aside from that big chip on my shoulder, my training was going well, my body was in near perfect condition and even the local newspaper promised the community that I, Sean Robbins, would make the team this time.

Setbacks are Inevitable

In my career, I have learned that physical setbacks will arise unexpectedly. Despite taking precautions and using well-planned training procedures, I strained a muscle while practicing a simple long jump drill that I had completed flawlessly every other time.

Imagine that you are driving to the most important meeting of your life and you blow a tire halfway there. You call for help or fix the tire---whatever it takes to get there, albeit late, out of breath and nervous.

That's kind of how I felt as I continued my workout program as the Olympic Trials date loomed closer. The last three weeks were the most challenging. I could barely sprint, much less jump, without suffering a bout of excruciating pain. But, by this time, my family and friend support team had already booked their flights to Sacramento, so there was no chance that I would forfeit. I was playing through the pain.

Missing the Mark

I arrived early on the field to prep for the long jump qualifying round. There were 24 jumpers competing, each with three attempts. Placement in the top 12 would earn a place in the finals two days later.

The energy from my fellow jumpers helped build my excitement and confidence during warm-ups. Got some high-fives, fist bumps and some hand claps. Trainers wrapped my leg up and I was as good as I was going to be. I almost forgot about my injury as I pushed on as planned.

Robbins up, Walder on deck, Phillips in the hole.

Nerves going crazy, I made my approach. 1..2..3..4..5..6..7...I counted my steps as I ran to keep my rhythm. I jumped and then... OUCH! The board judge held up the white flag, which meant it was a legal jump. 24 feet 1 inch. Nowhere near my best but I was happy to get a legal jump in my condition.

The next two jumps were made in severe pain and were accompanied by the judge's red flag (foul). Not the triumphant Nollywood or Bollywood ending that I had imagined earlier that summer.

I made a choice to continue through the pain at the trials. I did not want to disappoint my family and friends, but I also did not want to let myself down.

I have learned that things happen for a reason and it may be a while before we know the reason. I went to Sacramento knowing that only a miracle from GOD would get me on the team. When it was all over, I accepted my loss as another learning experience.

Facing Physical Setbacks

There will be setbacks in your training. Perhaps not as extreme as the experience I just recounted, but there are many factors in play that can slow (or sit) you down unexpectedly.

The key is being aware of your physical limitations in the event of a setback. Consult your physician or trainer to find out what you can do to avoid stopping your training completely, if possible. If you do have to take time off, make sure you have what you need to pick up where you left off, making any necessary adjustments.

You can go through, over or around a physical challenge---you still win as long as you get to the other side.

CAUSE AND EFFECT

Things will happen to impact your training---both positively and negatively. The trick is being aware of your body's normal functions and recognizing when something is not quite right.

Sometimes when you are working out, odd things might happen. You may feel a slight tinge of pain in your foot. A sharp pain in your shoulder. Maybe, a muscle pull in your leg. Or, one day you might feel great physically, in a good mood, and with endurance off the charts. Other days you may feel tired, with no motivation to even put on your training shoes. The good news is that many times, you might be able to pinpoint the cause of your issue.

I traveled to many countries during my professional track and field career. It might seem glamorous or exciting, but truthfully, as an athlete I had to be flexible because most of what I did was decided by someone else. Where I competed, the hotels I slept in, and sometimes even the food I ate. A trip to Stuttgart, Germany would require more flexibility than usual.

I was in Stuttgart for a few days, staying at a historic hotel. Like most cities in Europe at that time, businesses in Stuttgart closed at 6 p.m. Even the front desk of the hotel shut down, with the only English-speaking employee leaving to go home. With only Deutsch-speaking employees around, I used a lot of sign language after 6 p.m.

On Wednesday morning, one of the local coaches, Jonas, gave me a ride down to the practice track. It was a short drive, maybe less than 10 minutes. I chatted with Jonas while we drove through town past rows of historic look-alike buildings. I worked out for a few hours and was then ready to go back to the hotel for lunch and a nap.

Jonas was working with his group and suggested that I could walk back to the hotel. "It is right up the road." Since I had not paid enough attention to my surroundings on the way there, I decided to try to wait for Jonas. I had not packed any snacks that day so it was not long past my usual lunch hour before my stomach started notifying me that it was well past time to eat another meal. Five hours after breakfast. It was time to walk back to the hotel.

If you have ever walked through Stuttgart, or another old European city, you have noticed the beautiful architecture. That day, all I noticed was that everything looked the same as I walked and walked, staying parallel with the train tracks, the only landmark I was certain of. I ended up downtown, and after almost two hours, I decided to turn around and walk back in the direction I came from (nearly 7 hours without food). I probably should have stopped and asked for help. There had to be someone who might have spoken English. However, in my hungry state, I was not thinking clearly.

I reached my hotel around 6:00 p.m., past American dinner time (over 8 hours since my last meal). I was desperate for food at that late hour so I ate some local cuisine from a food truck. It was not the best dinner but I could not be choosy. Ugh. Time to get some sleep. Stuttgart exploration and adventure day---done.

The next day I went back to the practice track, this time making sure I knew how to get back to the hotel. I also packed some crackers and fruit, just in case.

During my workout, I was not feeling that great, and unfortunately, I pulled my hip flexor muscle. I was pretty sure that my adventures the day before had something to do with it.

Look for Changes

Changes to your sleep cycle, work routine, training plan, diet or meal schedule can often lead to undesired results. In my case, the causes of my bad day on the track were obvious---all of the unplanned walking, and hours of not eating the previous day had an immediate effect on my performance. I was not able to train at my normal level.

Consider these common causes for weakness, pain, or other discomfort.

- Overdoing it. An example might be going from running a 20-minute mile one day and trying to do it in 10 minutes the next. Or, doing bicep curls with 35-pound weights, instead of the normal 20-pound weights. It would be more beneficial to use a gradual approach to increasing intensity or weight.

- Food and drink changes. A few cups of coffee to stay awake after a late night at the bar. Trying a new dish or eating at a new restaurant. Forgetting to drink enough water. These changes may not seem significant, but most people will notice a difference, especially if they have disciplined eating habits. Pay attention to what you eat and bring extra water when you work out.

- Changes to medicines and supplements. Noticeable changes can occur after taking a new medication or stopping an existing medication. Use caution by communicating with your medical professional about your exercise program before starting, stopping, or changing a medication.

- Travel. Traveling by air or taking long road trips can affect circulation. Going to higher elevations may cause headaches. Visiting places unknown with different air quality, water and food choices beyond their control affects people differently, and can have short-term, and sometimes long-term, impacts on health and wellness. Be proactive and make a plan to prevent you from having to take a vacation after your vacation.

Track Changes

Keep a log or notebook listing what you eat and drink, your physical activities, hours of sleep and any interruptions. Note any unusual aftereffects. This will help you to stay aware of any health changes and identify potential causes. Although you may not get to the root cause of every negative effect, keeping good notes will often help you and your medical professional to pinpoint triggers.

DOMINO EFFECT

"I really didn't know what I was doing. I had watched others using the machine but I must have turned or lifted wrong because I felt something pop in my right shoulder. It did not hurt immediately but over a few weeks, I started to notice the twinge of pain more and more when I worked out. I stopped doing the lifting exercise and so my shoulder would only hurt once in a while, and only if I lifted something heavy.

I bought a protective sling, used smaller weights and so I thought the intermittent pain would eventually pass. Instead, I found that I could not lift my right arm past a certain level without pain. The next time I attempted to play basketball, I fell on the floor writhing in pain after I grabbed a rebound. I was done. My doctor diagnosed me with 'frozen shoulder' (adhesive capsulitis). Without surgery, it took over a year of rehab to be able to reach both arms straight over my head."

Fix Your Injury or Else: Effects of an injury left unchecked

Addressing an injury from the start is the most important thing you can do to sustain your training. When you are doing an exercise and you feel a tweak, or sharp pain, your mind might lead you to "*Keep going!*" but your body might be screaming, "*Stop, just stop!*" If you decide to listen to both voices, you will meet in the middle and compromise to go slower. Regardless of the intensity of the pain you feel after an injury, and no matter how often you feel the pain, you have to address it.

During one of my track meets, I slightly sprained my right Achilles tendon---a jumper's nightmare injury. I rested, did therapy, and adjusted my training exercises to give myself time to heal. After a few weeks, I felt ready to get going again.

The next time I did sprint drills with the sprain, I actually felt pretty good. Did I feel it? Yes, I definitely felt it a little, but after all the time I had taken off from sprinting, I was happy to just be able to do it.

Fast forward a few more weeks of still feeling that tinge, trying to go easy on it, but pushing myself more and more to get back to my full performance. What I did not realize was, all that time I was going easy on my right side, I was putting extra pressure on my left knee and hip. I did not become fully aware of it until I started feeling pain in my left side hip and knee. Even though I was addressing the original Achilles injury, my body was not quite ready for me to sprint. I fell victim to what I call the ***injury domino effect***.

We must take care to address all injuries, even if we believe that they are minor. They can linger and become major injuries or affect other parts of the body. Healing and recovery take time, so be patient. Remember that repairing the original injury, however minor it may seem, will lead to the gains you want in your training.

GPS: Reroute Your Injury

Have you ever been driving in an unfamiliar area and needed to rely on your GPS? If you miss a turn, or go the wrong way, the GPS pauses and a spinning circle appears. That lets you know that it's working, recalculating, and loading a new driving plan for you. Very soon it emits those pleasant words that comfort you and let you know that you are not lost: "Rerouting...Rerouting."

One of the biggest challenges a personal trainer faces is motivating clients to continue their training when injuries occur. Rather than ending the training, I help them reroute their training plan, adapting to a temporary change.

I worked with a client who sprained her ankle while playing tennis. Her first thought was to take time off from training. Instead of taking the week off, she trained through her injury. With her ankle immobile, she worked out on the fly machine, did lat pulls and sitting battle ropes, and other exercises that did not apply pressure to her ankle.

Typically, you might think that an ankle injury would shut down your training program but instead, it should only reroute you like the GPS when you make a wrong turn. Rerouting your vehicle may mean taking a U-turn, going through an area you are not familiar with or driving a lot further than you planned, delaying your ETA. Rerouting your training means taking time and getting some extra help.

Your recovery from an injury may determine whether you will be able to continue to do certain exercises in the future. If you are an athlete, an injury may determine when you retire from a sport. Getting professional training assistance will help you navigate a training plan even with a brace, cast, sling, bandage, and/or crutches.

There are several hundred muscle groups and joints in the body.

There are many variations of exercises that you can perform while avoiding your injured area.

How do you determine when you are past your injury? Typically, there will be some muscle soreness but, for most:

- It will not hurt during the exercise.
- It will not hurt after the exercise, or later in the day.
- It will not hurt the next day.
- Your medical professional will clear you.

Rerouting your workout means different things depending on the type of injury and your overall physical condition. The concept is simple: do not allow your injury to stop your workout---just reroute it and get help from a training professional if necessary.

SEAN ROBBINS

Shortcuts & Fads

ENTERTAINMENT FITNESS

Social media shines a light on exercise and fitness in a number of ways. Some encourage people to get active and demonstrate standard exercises. For others, the purpose is to get attention. I refer to those videos as entertainment fitness.

The same characteristics that make any social media post go viral also apply to fitness videos. Those that show someone doing standard exercises, such as bench-pressing weights or running on a treadmill will not capture much attention; however, seeing someone hanging upside down and doing bicep curls, or running or jogging through a high-traffic or otherwise dangerous environment will get the desired clicks.

Unusual and Entertaining

People like to post exercises that are different and challenging. Different does not always mean it's a good choice and challenging does not always mean the activity will be beneficial.

Now, I agree that it looks cool to see people walking up steps while balancing on their hands. However, I have not watched a handstand stair climbing tournament, and, although Simone Biles would probably sign up, it is not (yet) an Olympic event. Recognize the difference between beneficial exercise and just entertainment fitness.

Here are some examples of some challenges you might encounter:

- Weight loss challenge
- Obstacle course challenge
- Plank challenge
- Step running challenge

Fitness challenges are fun, motivating and an excellent method to build teams and bond with others through group exercise. The question we all must ask is whether a particular challenge is appropriate for us. Before signing up, find out who will facilitate the challenge. Will someone demonstrate proper technique and form of the required exercises or activities, and also explain the benefits? Is that person certified or otherwise qualified to lead the challenge (a trainer, coach, athlete, etc.)? Is the location conducive to the planned activities? Ensure that you are comfortable with these aspects in advance of joining. Know whether it is right or wrong for you.

Challenges Have Deadlines

Fitness challenges are short-term, time-limited activities. For many, it is an excellent way to start on the fitness journey. When the challenge ends, do not stop there. Move beyond the challenge to training, keeping in mind that some fitness challenge activities can definitely be integrated into a long-term, balanced training program.

Balanced Training

Some training is designed to excite and entertain for a short period of time. Different does not necessarily mean better. The best type of training is long-term, consisting of varied exercises and corresponds to individual capabilities. Long-term training suits those seeking to Play Long and Stay Strong. Entertainment fitness is, well, entertaining. Recognize the difference.

ENTERTAINMENT SPORTS

Saturday afternoons at home are often spent clicking through the TV or streaming channels to find a sports competition. We especially enjoy watching BMX riders and skateboarders fling themselves into the air, soar across barriers and seemingly miraculously land upright. I hold my breath watching Parkour athletes jump, flip, and roll without stopping to check whether a bone fractured on the last landing.

Those athletes train for the high-risk sports and are conditioned for their highly entertaining---and often dangerous---performances. No matter the sport, if it is something new, be sure to get the training and conditioning necessary before jumping into it. Before getting involved in a new activity, be aware of your individual capabilities and stay safe.

Stick With the Fist Bump

The final point on the topic of entertainment sports applies to casual, amateur, and professional athletes alike: take it easy on the celebrations.

When someone blocks a shot or scores a goal it is natural to want to celebrate with a fist bump, a high-five, a muscle flex or even a dance move. All in good fun but beyond that, athletes are injuring themselves while celebrating. The knee slides across the soccer field grass resulting in torn ligaments. High flying chest bumps on the basketball court ending with head injuries. Front and back flips on the football field leaving players with sprains. Human pile-ups that sideline athletes for weeks. Entertainment sport can involve incidental damages. At any level of sport, slapping a hand or two definitely does not hurt as much.

It all comes down to this: play your sport and stay safe while doing it. Leave the thrill-seeking to the professionals and when you make that great play, smile, nod, and act like it's not the first time you did it. Your body will thank you.

ENTERTAINMENT DIET

Have you ever noticed how many people are so-called experts in diet and health? Or at least they want to be. When it comes to diet, always consider your goals and your individual nutritional needs.

Extreme Weight Changes

Celebrities use their fame to promote and share their healthy lifestyles. Part of their appeal is the combination of good looks, fit bodies, perfect attire, and sparkling smiles---all honed for magazine and social media perfection. Although they normally attempt to retain that appearance at all times, there are times that they change their looks deliberately.

At times, actors gain weight for movie roles and then appear a few months later having returned to their normal size. When Will Smith was interviewed about the movie, "Ali," he described how he packed on 30 pounds of muscle for his highly acclaimed role as Muhammad Ali. He also packed on the pounds to become the genie in Aladdin, as did Tom Hanks, Viola Davis, and Charlize Theron for their movie roles. It takes discipline, dedication, and a great deal of willpower to later lose the weight. Most of us know from personal experience that losing weight takes a lot longer than gaining it.

One of my previous clients, whom I will call Sally, was very upfront at our first meeting. She said, with a very serious expression on her face, "Sean, I need to train with you for three months to get ready for my school reunion. I have to lose 25 pounds so I need your best diet and exercise plan."

I just looked at her, nodded and smiled an understanding smile. She was not the first (and would not be the last) to believe that she had the time, stamina, and willpower to "go Hollywood" with her weight loss and fitness goals.

I asked Sally, "Well, how much time do you have?" That question opened up a discussion about the amount of time that she would need to exercise, and about what she would need to eat (or not eat) daily to meet her deadline. My questions changed her perspective and allowed her to think more realistically about what was achievable.

My next question was really a showstopper. "What are your plans after you make your school reunion appearance?" That discussion was about whether she planned to continue to train, or just get as fit as possible, attend the reunion, and then go back to whatever she was doing previously. When considering entertainment diets people usually do not think past their deadlines.

In Sally's case, she trained with me, went to her reunion, came back, and continued working with me. Long story short, we ended up training together for eight years. There's a saying: *If you're already ready then you don't have to get ready.* That is, being ready for reunions, weddings, beach vacations, photo shoots and work---and any other occasions and places where people want to look their best---means getting in shape and staying in shape, whatever that means for the individual. Needless to say, once she started training regularly, Sally was always ready for all of her important events and occasions.

Quick Fixes

Detoxification is an unfortunate and necessary medical treatment for anyone who has consumed chemicals, ingested poisons, or other hazardous substances. Dietary detoxing is one of the popular approaches to losing weight and what is referred to as a cleansing. This trendy method reportedly clears the body of impurities, toxins, and other unhealthy things that a person has eaten or drunk.

Detoxing is an extreme entertainment diet and involves eliminating what is considered unhealthy---fatty, sugary, and processed foods---and eating or drinking what is considered healthy---fruits, vegetables, and *clean* foods. Dietary detoxing can also restrict mobility because it may require staying at home, close to the bathroom.

When it comes to food and drink, if we eat healthy and drink healthy every day, then there is no need to detoxify. Adding fruits and vegetables like apples, melons, broccoli, asparagus, kale, and other greens to your meals will do the detoxing duty on a daily basis--and no one has to stay at home all day.

A Diet that Works

A healthy diet is not temporary; it relies on ongoing healthy choices, not quick fixes. Plan and implement a balanced and sustainable diet of nutritious foods and avoid entertainment diets that lead to weight fluctuations or deprivation.

The diet that works for you is created with your health needs, schedule, and fitness goals in mind. The diet that works is all about you.

ENTERTAINMENT EQUIPMENT

"Only five minutes a day on the body fat presser and I lost 25 pounds in just two weeks!"

Now if that machine actually existed (and it does not, by the way), would you buy it? Would you be so excited by those claims that you would call or go online to make a purchase? Many people do indeed purchase what I refer to as entertainment equipment---fitness equipment that seems too good to be true, and most of the time it is. What's worse, is after the novelty wears off, the equipment often gets pushed to a corner, a closet, or the curbside of a house when it does not live up to its exaggerated benefits.

Sometimes the entertainment equipment infomercials are so believable, anyone might be lured into buying, even athletes. When I coached at Ashland University, one of our best athletes took the bait and fell into the trap.

One afternoon, a promising high jumper came to track practice with more than the normal pep in his step; in fact, it looked like he was prancing. He seemed taller---about three inches taller. I looked down at his feet and saw that he was wearing some highly advertised, trendy athletic shoes, the kind designed to elevate the front portion of the foot for the purpose of strengthening the calf muscles. I was very familiar with the shoes. The TV and magazine ads claimed that the shoes would *help you run faster and jump higher*. Perhaps they could, but they were quite a sight.

"Coach Sean, I want to practice in these." Pause. While I stared at him, I considered requiring him to change into his regular practice shoes. But instead of making an equipment change mandate, I decided that it would be a good day for him to learn a lesson.

The jumpers' workout consisted of 100-meter sprints, plyometrics over hurdles, and some hill runs. Towards the end of practice my jumper kept rubbing his lower legs. When I asked how he was feeling, he grimaced and answered, "My calves are on fire!" I said to him calmly, "Just stretch them out and I'll see you at practice tomorrow." I watched him as he limped off the track and down the hill to the team facility.

The next day there was no prancing---only limping. The good news was, he was not wearing those designer shoes. The bad news was, he was still suffering from some calf muscle soreness. The teaching moment had arrived.

I acknowledged the well-intentioned attempts to improve his jumping abilities but explained that using those specially made shoes would not give him the results he wanted. The shoe was designed to increase the force on his calf muscles but that was unnecessary *(and unnatural)* because he was already training his calves by performing the drills and exercises at practice. There was no need to use equipment---on in this case special shoes---that focused solely on the calves. He nodded and retired the shoes.

A few months later when my jumper placed 2nd at the NCAA National meet, he understood that his success was due to a balanced training program. It was not the shoes.

More Than Meets the Eye

Thigh muscle burners, electronic abdominal muscle twitch activators, animated equipment, freezing or super hot enclosures, and trendy clothing and shoes---the list is long. The marketers tell us that using their products will help us to achieve our sports and fitness goals in 15-minutes a day. Remember to read the fine print. Whether or not you can actually read the fine print on the screen, that 15-minutes of use must be accompanied by a healthy diet and other daily exercises before you will see any changes.

So, do not be tricked when you see the extremely fit, ripped, or toned person demonstrating the machine. That body was chiseled well before that new product was even designed. Also, do not be enticed by the before and after photos. Yes, the spray tans make them look thinner and yes, that guy is sucking in his gut in the after photo.

Getting fit takes time and effort. Playing long and staying strong is not done in 15-minutes per day. Rather than buying equipment that only focuses on your calves, abs, or any particular body part or muscle group, buy a membership to a fitness center where you can work out your entire body. Using entertainment equipment alone will not work, so save your money and leave the magic machines on the shelf.

Tips for Your Training Journey

SELF-IMPOSED LIMITATIONS

I am really out of shape.
I don't have time to do this.
I'm not motivated.
I don't have a gym membership.
I'm too old for this.

Make a list of 50 excuses for not moving forward with any activity and I am willing to bet that I have heard all of them before from my clients. Those listed above are my top five. Did you know that none of them come with a doctor's note?

Getting Past the "No" in Your Head

One of my clients, Trisha, began training with me in her early 50s. She trusted me enough to help her get into shape but balked when I explained the training plan. When I told her that she would be doing sprints, she protested, "But I have not done sprints since my 20s! I'm slow and too old!"

I chuckled and told her that since I was not training her for the Olympics, that I would only be recording her running speed for use in creating her training plan and tracking her progress. It would also be a way to challenge her stamina a bit. She did not seem convinced by the rationale, but she agreed to go along with it.

The first few days at the outdoor track were not great. Trisha struggled some with the A-Skip, B-Skip and Low-knees drills, but I attributed some of that to her nervousness. She was outside her comfort zone and like anyone, it affected her performance.

However, it was not long before she became more at ease and improved. She learned the drills and was doing them correctly, at her own pace. The best day of training was the day that she saw a group of high school track athletes doing the same drills, and she pointed out the students who were doing them incorrectly. Her awareness of the drill, and her ability to assess others as a coach would, indicated that both her knowledge and confidence were growing.

Never Too Young

One of the younger clients I worked with was an 11-year-old named Sidney. Sidney's mother told me that he was thrilled to start training, mainly because he was tired of ending up in last place when his basketball team ran sprints at practice.

On our first day of training together, I asked Sidney to run one lap around the track. Before I had the chance to finish telling him what to do, Sidney took off running in a blaze of fury, and using the most awful running form.

He was breathing hard when he completed his lap and could barely stand up. "That was supposed to be your warm up lap," I told him. He nodded. "Yes. I'm warm now." I laughed and told him that there was more to the warm-up, specifically stretching. "Stretching? I don't need to stretch. I'm ready!"

At his age, understandably, Sidney had a misconception about the need to stretch. Like some adults, he did not think it was necessary. I demonstrated a few stretching exercises and Sidney did them dutifully, and with a bored look on his face. "Why do I need to do so many stretches?" It was a good opening for the teaching moment that came next.

I explained to Sidney that stretching kept his muscles strong and flexible. As he grew older, he would develop more muscles and stretching would ensure that his muscles would continue to be loose and flexible. And, I explained further, he would continue to be able to run when he was older.

He kind of stared blankly at me. I did not think he was appreciating the value of the information I was providing so finally, I said, "Stretching your muscles is like brushing your teeth. You never feel like doing it but someday you'll be very unhappy if you don't." I think he got it then.

Never Too Old

Never think that you are too young to start making better or new choices for your health and fitness, and never believe that you are too old to do that either.

Before you say "yes" or "no" to an activity or exercise, make sure your reasons are valid for why you should or should not try it---and your age is not always a valid reason. However, your physical capabilities are different from those of others so be self-aware before choosing an activity. You can always focus more time and attention on the activities that you are capable of doing.

They've Still Got It!

Have you ever watched the Senior Olympics? Search for videos online and prepare to be amazed. Those 50 and older athletes look just as good as their younger counterparts. Well, of course they are in top physical condition if they are competing in the Olympics.

The point is this: they choose to continue to train and compete in a sport they enjoy, despite their advanced age, and they avoid anything that might sound like an excuse.

Training to climb Mt. Everest in the senior years is not for everyone but Yuchiro Miura did it at 80 years old. No matter where you are in life, there is an activity for you. Don't knock it until you've tried it!

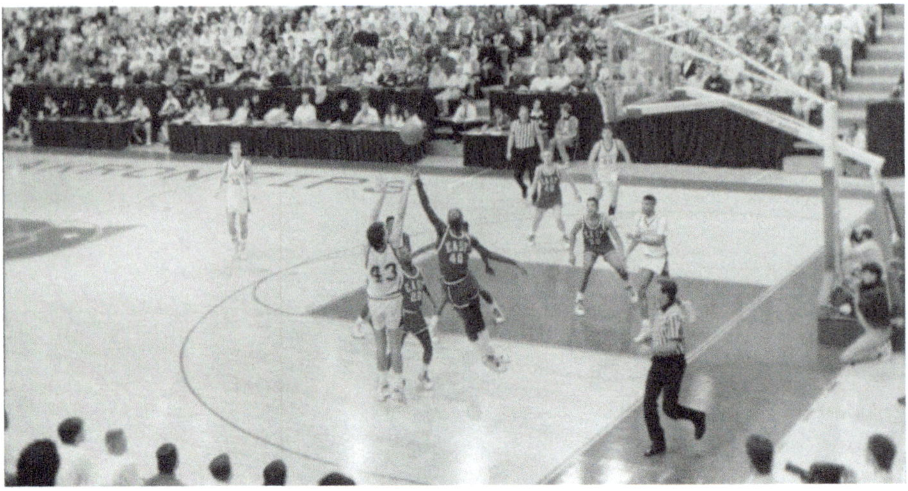

PLAYING WITH YOUR PEERS

Think back to when you were a kid. Most of us have fond memories of learning in school, playing sports, and advancing as we grew older. We were grouped according to our age, grade and/or skill level to make sure we fit in with our peers.

Growing up, I had the good fortune of living across the street from a park and recreation center. My parents planned that well because they always knew where I was. They knew I was safe and that I would always be on time for dinner.

I spent many hours at Joy Park after school and on weekends. I looked forward to the day camp program that was held at the park during the summer break. The camp program was like a job for me. I was up and out at 7:30 a.m. and finished up at 4:30 p.m.

On the first day of camp, the counselors conducted an orientation. The camp director sat us all down and announced the rules, regulations, and the consequences of not following the rules and regulations. After they indoctrinated us, the crowd of kids was separated into groups of boys and girls, and then further divided into camp teams by age.

"Ages 7 to 9, raise your hands. Go to Carter." Carter stood smiling, waiting for his group. "Ages 10 to 12, head to Jacobs." As I was about to raise my hand and head over, one of my older friends grabbed my arm and kept it down. Mike gave me a look that I quickly interpreted as, "Stay here." Still holding my arm, he whispered, "You're going to be in our group."

"Ages 13 to 15, go to Williams." Mike nudged me and off I went with my friends to join Mr. Williams, a tall man with a broad smile and a loud, booming voice. When I settled in with the group, one of the assistants looked at me and said, "How old are you? Are you sure you are in the right group?" Mike looked over and blurted out, "Yes, he's our age!" Another good friend backed him up. "He's 13!" During those years, we did not have any IDs so the words of two (false) witnesses were apparently enough to clear me. (*Lord forgive me for the lie...*)

Playing Above Your Level

I was officially part of the group made up of my neighborhood friends and the older boys, and I was ready to get going with all the activities. We played dodgeball, basketball, football and tennis. We even played softball---and I was terrible at it. I was very athletic but since I had not hit the growth spurt yet to come, playing with the older boys meant I got pushed around and plowed over sometimes. Most of them were better and faster than me but they pushed me (literally and physically) to improve as I attempted to keep up with them. Despite the challenges, playing above my level at an early age was helpful to me in future years, particularly in track and basketball.

Playing with people more advanced than you has its benefits, if you can keep up. One of my younger clients, a tennis player, became really good at tennis when he competed against older kids. Now that he is older, he is a top player. The players in his age group play slightly below his level so now he has to look beyond his field of peers to find competitors at a higher level. Better competitors can push you to play at your highest level and winning---or getting close---will further build your confidence.

Playing At Your Level

My experience playing with older kids built my confidence and skill level. Now that I am older, I am still playing basketball with other men and boys of various ages. This time, however, I am the older guy and I am still hanging in there with the younger guys as I stay in shape and continue to play.

Sometimes at my gym, I watch a group of men 60 and older playing basketball. I admire their stamina and ability, and I think to myself, I hope that I will have the ability to play basketball at that age.

As I observe them, I notice that they move somewhat slower, but they still have a level of agility that works for their level of the game. Regardless of how fast they move, they can all shoot the lights out. Most of the players in this group compete in major senior tournaments. They are skilled players and the key is that they were all playing at their level of ability.

I talked with one of the players and asked what motivated him to keep playing basketball, even at the risk of injuring himself. I knew that he had knee issues and had undergone at least two surgeries. He smiled and explained that he stayed in the game purely for the enjoyment of the sport, and he only played with people at his skill level. He knew exactly how fast he could run.

The group often reserves the basketball court for only 60 and over players. The explanation given to any members who complained was that it was for the safety of the senior players. By only playing with their peers, these guys stay healthy and minimize the risk of injury.

Play Where You Fit In

Depending on where you are in life, you may be playing or training with people who are older, younger or the same age as you. Your peer group is made up of the people who are at your physical level. Get to know your capabilities and limitations and play where you fit in. *Age ain't nothing but a number* but mature bones heal slowly.

SEAN ROBBINS

Keeping it together

ADJUSTING TO PHYSICAL CHANGES OVER TIME

As much as we like to think that *we've still got it*, after reaching a certain age, we only have some of it left. By our 40s, most of us are at a lower level than we were in our 20s or even 30s. Accepting that reality is important to understanding current capabilities.

Recognize that although you are no longer in your 20s, that does not mean that you cannot do what you did when you were in your 20s. As you age, you just have to adjust what you do and how you do it. The preparation for your sport or activity is different than it was before. The duration you play is different. What you eat and drink have to be different.

When I retired from track and field, I set a personal goal to continue to do as much training as I did when I was competing. No, I did not intend to continue to actually jump in the sand, but I did continue my sprinting, plyometrics, and power lifts so I have been able to maintain that goal rather successfully. Every once in a while, I get a question about whether I am still competing. *Yeah, (I look like) I've still got it.*

Like me, you too can continue to train. You may not do plyometrics, but you have plenty of options. As mentioned previously, getting to know your physical capabilities helps determine what you can do. Whatever that is, do it to its fullest.

Know Your History

Part of understanding our physical capabilities is understanding our genes and family medical histories. This is important at every stage, but especially as we age. We need to know what is happening with our health to adjust how we train or vary the sports we play.

Researching family history can reveal potential conditions and illnesses like high blood pressure, a condition that is prevalent in my family. To address it, I take the preventive measure of reducing salt intake. For others, a family history of arthritis or heart conditions might be concerns. Whatever the health issues *might* be, the only way to be certain is to schedule and show up for medical exams. No surprises.

DOING THE WORK

Yes. You. Can.

Believing in yourself and your ability to accomplish what you seek to do is essential for athletes of all types. Each time they walk on a court, field, or course, or dive into a pool to compete, they have faith that they will win.

As a man of faith, I especially enjoy sharing my knowledge and experiences with others. I have done many presentations in churches on physical training and its benefits. In that environment, the discussion often turns to the impacts of prayer and faith on a person's health. Both are known to be positive factors in healing and recovery. I believe in both faith and prayer as powerful complements to hard work.

Faith Without Physical Works

I had the pleasure of training my former church pastor for nearly a year. During our sessions, he shared the many challenges he faced as a pastor. He said that he often prayed for his members and their various health and physical concerns. He recognized that most often, prayer accompanied by action was more effective than prayer alone.

As believers, we pray for the health conditions and needs of others. Any requests for prayer should be granted. As a trainer---*if it is appropriate for the condition*---I take it one step further by asking the person what actions she or he is taking to assist healing and recovery. That is the question I asked when I conducted my fitness and wellness presentation for my fellow church members. Pastor's response: an invitation to all church members to join him on a daily morning walk.

Nobody Likes to do Push-Ups

No one likes to do push-ups, but everyone wants the lean, muscular pecs, deltoids, triceps, and arms that they produce. You have to put in the work to get the results you want from your training. Have faith in yourself to achieve, make a plan and implement it. Now drop and give me 25! 1...2...3...

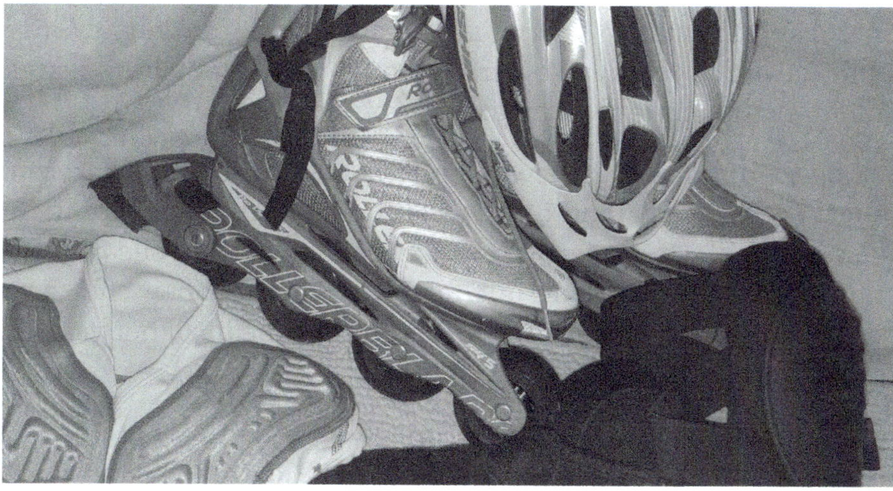

ROLLING THROUGH THE YEARS

I can always tell when the weather is really warm and that spring has truly arrived. It happens on the first morning that my wife Cheryl gets up and out "before the cars start rolling," to skate or bike in the neighborhood.

Cheryl has been skating for a LONG time. I am not permitted to tell you how old she is, but she has been skating most of her life. She skated as a child, four-wheel quad skates in rinks and in her neighborhood. In college she tried ice skating (too cold) but fell in love with inline skating. She spent some birthday gift money on some Rollerblades instead of spending a night out getting her first legal drinks. She found some like-minded friends and she has been rolling ever since, mostly alone these days.

I enjoy skating too---quads, not rollerblades. For a few years,

Cheryl and I would go skating at a local rink on adult night, when adult meant 15 years and older. We bought some matching skates, but I drew the line at wearing matching clothing.

Cheryl upgraded to newer Rollerblades on her most recent milestone birthday (and I think she has started pre-shopping for the next one). On a recent Saturday morning, she yelled up the stairs that she was going out for a short roll. When she came back, she told me that she fell for the third time in all her years of rollerblading.

She did not look to be broken anywhere and I thought that she had come into the house and was telling me all this right after she fell down. Instead, she described how she got her skate caught in a driveway crevice, tripped and fell, got up and washed herself off with the hose, and then rolled off to continue her morning skate.

The fall could have been more damaging but Cheryl has always worn protective gear---knee pads, safety glasses, elbow pads, helmet, wrist guards---and is generally careful about where and when she skates. She recognizes that as she ages, safety becomes even more important.

Make sure you take safety into account as you age and continue playing your sport or participating in physical activities. Fortunately, Cheryl only scraped her shoulder. Her last comment about it was, "I have to buy some shoulder pads now."

CAREER LONGEVITY

If you are a professional athlete, you have to train and perfect your performance for a long-lasting career. As a coach, I have to continue to stay on top of my game in order to train others. Similarly, health professionals, retail workers, restaurant waitstaff, warehouse employees, office staff, construction and other industry professionals also need to train for the physical requirements that it takes to do their jobs well.

Your level of physical fitness will determine how well you can "compete" in your daily activities---whether the job involves sitting and typing at a desk, standing for long periods, lifting, bending, turning, or frequent walking. All jobs have a physical component.

Many progressive companies have added fitness facilities, healthier dining options and wellness programs to change their workforce culture. They have added financial incentives to keeping their employees on the job and incurring fewer medical care and insurance costs. Their goal is to minimize, or eliminate completely, the common work-related ailments that affect their bottom lines. Not all companies offer wellness benefits to their employees, and for the ones that do, well workforce programs work best when there are facilitators and trainers to guide participants.

Traditionally, professional athletes have coaches and trainers to help them to hone their bodies and perfect their performance. They also have access to all the equipment that they need and personnel to support their training. Professionals in other fields of work could use a little support, too.

Regardless of the profession, all organizations can benefit from improving the health of their employees. Workers who have access to fitness trainers, and along with onsite equipment, will benefit from the efforts to impact their health and longevity. One of my goals is to demonstrate that even simple physical routines will improve worker performance.

"Play Long Stay Strong." is a mindset, as well as guidance for improving sports, fitness, and wellness both now and in the future, to ensure that you can keep doing what you enjoy for the long haul.

Lifelong training is not always easy. It is up to you to do the work. It takes discipline, time management and commitment to stay in the game.

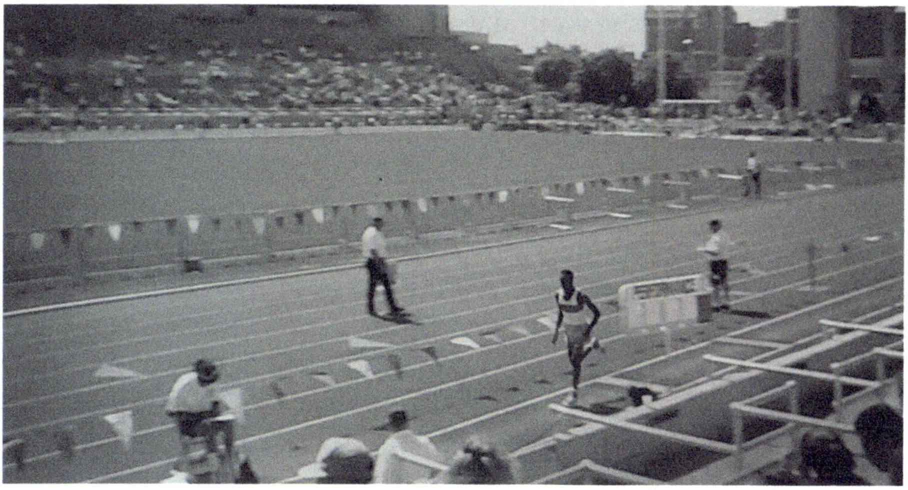

FIND YOUR LONG JUMP SUCCESS

When I was a kid, basketball was the most popular sport. I saw it played everywhere from TV to the park across the street. So, in the first year in junior high, my close friends and I tried out for the basketball team.

At tryouts, we were all rather confident that we would make the team. My goal was to do everything I could to impress the coach: I made my free-throws, lay-ups, an occasional jump shot and a few steals. But all of my hoop dreams came crashing down when I could not do the three-man weave.

The three-man weave drill puts your true basketball skills on full display and when you mess up, everybody can see it. My inability to do the drill prevented me from making the basketball team.

Aghrrr. The salt in the wound was that year, the players that made the cut went undefeated for the season. At school, everyone called them "Super 6." (Personally, I think "Super 7" would have sounded a whole lot better.)

Getting cut from the basketball team was a tough break but it did not knock me off my athletic quest; it only pushed me to try another sport. So that same year I tried out for wrestling. Heck, I thought, what's so hard about pinning your opponent on his back? I had watched WWF on television and I knew all the moves. It turned out that wrestling was a bit harder than I thought, especially given the fact that my opponent was trying to pin me down, too. That was a short, four-week long wrestling career. Aghrrr again.

Finally, I decided to try my luck running track. Looking for a way to redeem myself from recent failures, I was certain this one had to work out. Track and field has many events and I figured that between the track sprinting and hurdling, and the field jumping and throwing, there had to be something that I could do, and do well. Let's do this!

The good news was I made the team. Success! After making the team, my next step was to figure out which event(s) I would do. The event that most of us kids wanted to do was the 100-meter dash, and I was decent
enough to compete in it. The coach saw some potential in me and asked me to compete in the 110 hurdles and the high jump events as well.

"Sure, Coach." It could not be that hard sprinting 110 meters and jumping over 10 lined up fences. I could jump fences all day. Jumping backwards over a high stick did not seem to be much of a challenge either. Ok cool.

The coach, seeing that I did pretty well in the hurdles and high jump, asked me to try one more event--the long jump. I was not as thrilled about this event and the idea of getting sand everywhere on my body---and I do mean everywhere. On top of it all, I was not very good at it. But I stuck with it anyway.

I kept practicing and, surprisingly, I became much better in the long jump than in the other events. It was then that I first discovered my long jump success.

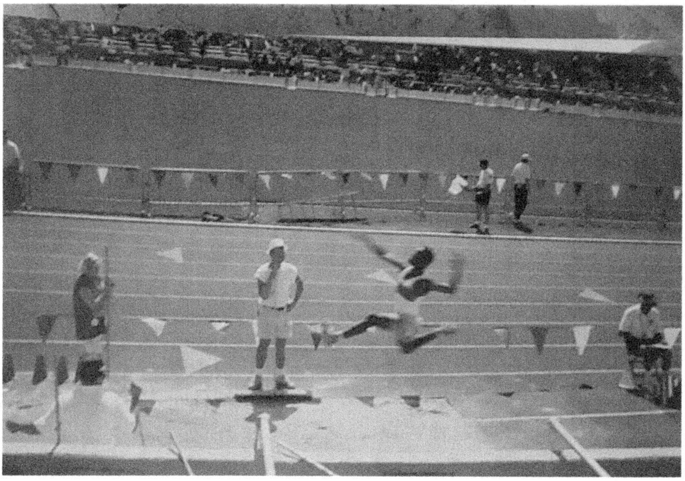

Exposure Matters

Many times, the lack of exposure to the universe of sports or activities will prevent kids from finding something they are good at doing. If their goal is to play football or basketball---*but they cannot play either sport well*---then without intervention to guide them to other sports, they may not ever find their success in sports. I was fortunate because I did. The additional guidance of my coach helped me to think beyond basketball to find my place in track and field. (And by the way, I made the basketball team the next year because I became a master of the three-man weave.)

Some people are not suited to play all competitive sports or train in every exercise. As a trainer and coach, my job is to help clients to find their own version of success. I guide each person to find the most appropriate exercises or activities for getting started and then sustaining their training journeys---whether athletic or fitness.

Getting started is often the most difficult part of the journey. I coach clients through exercises that might seem impossible at first, or even exercises they do not want to do. However, with practice, conditioning, and consistency they are often impressed at their newfound capabilities. Even when things do not go well, they keep going anyway. There is a long jump out there for everyone. Find yours.

Play Long. Stay Strong.

ABOUT THE AUTHOR

Fitness & Sports Excellerated, LLC Lead Trainer, Coach Sean Robbins, is a former world-class athlete, fitness and wellness educator, professional speaker and author.

In Play Long. Stay Strong., Sean shares sports and fitness information important to starting and continuing a training program---and at any age.

Coach Sean operates FSE Fitness Studio, a fully equipped 2000 square foot fitness and training center in North Canton, Ohio, and he consults at other NE Ohio facilities.

Sean coached at Baker University and at Ashland University, his alma mater. He is currently a fitness and agility consultant for football officials in the Big 10, MAC, and Missouri Valley conferences. He also administers the assessment tests for officials in the NFL and the PAC 12 conference.

Contact Coach Sean by visiting:
www.PlayLongStayStrong.com

BIBLIOGRAPHY

How Dianne Durham, Bela Karolyi's first national champion, paved the way for Black gymnasts. Bonnie D. Ford and Alyssa Roenigk. July 18, 2021. https://www.espn.com/olympics/story/_/id/29469312/how-dianne-durham-bela-karolyi-first-national-champion-paved-way-black-gymnasts

Strug's Heart of Gold helps U.S. take top honors. Larry Schwartz. July 23, 1996. http://www.espn.com/classic/s/moment010723-strug-gold.html

Will Smith Gained Nearly 200 Pounds For His Role As Muhammad Ali In 'Ali'. Vaishnavi Navalka. August 9, 2020. https://www.republicworld.com/entertainment-news/hollywood-news/will-smith-gained-nearly-200-pounds-for-role-as-muhammad-ali-in-ali.html

80-year-old Yuichiro Miura claims new Everest record. Tom Bayly. May 23, 2013. https://www.bbc.com/news/av/world-asia-22644717

Made in the USA
Monee, IL
03 November 2026

67385924R00069